The REGENTS/PRENTICE HALL
MEDICAL ASSISTANT KIT

NEUROLOGY

Third Edition

REGENTS/PRENTICE HALL, Englewood Cliffs, New Jersey 07632

Library of Congress Cataloging-in-Publication Data
Neurology.— 3rd ed.
    p. cm.—(The Regents/Prentice Hall medical assistant kit)
    Rev. ed. of: Neurology/ [by Elizabeth K. White]. 2nd ed. c1985.
    Includes index.
    ISBN 0-13-036823-7
    1. Nervous system—Diseases. 2. Neurology. 3. Sense organs—
Diseases. 4. Allied health personnel. I. White, Elizabeth K.
Neurology. II. Regents/Prentice Hall. III. Series.
    [DNLM: 1. Neurology. WL 100 N494911]
    RC346.W49 1992
    616.8—dc20
    DNLM/DLC
    for Library of Congress   92-48848
                                                                   CIP

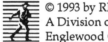
© 1993 by REGENTS/PRENTICE HALL
A Division of Simon & Schuster
Englewood Cliffs, NJ 07632

Notice
The information and procedures described in the REGENTS/PRENTICE HALL MEDICAL
ASSISTANT KIT are based on consultation with practitioners and instructors and are to be
used as part of a formal course taught by a qualified Medical Assistant instructor. To the
best of the publisher's knowledge, this information reflects currently accepted practices;
however, it cannot be considered absolute recommendations. For individual application,
the policies and procedures of the institution or agency where the Medical Assistant is
employed must be reviewed and followed. The authors of these materials and their supple-
ments disclaim responsibility for any adverse effects resulting directly or indirectly from
the suggested procedures and theory, from any undetected errors, or from the reader's
misunderstanding of the materials. It is the reader's responsibility to stay informed of any
new changes or recommendations made by his or her employing health care institution or
agency.

Printed in the United States of America

10 9 8 7 6 5 4 3 2 1

ISBN   0-13-0368237-7   NB2I

Prentice-Hall International (UK) Limited, *London*
Prentice-Hall of Australia Pty. Limited, *Sydney*
Prentice-Hall Canada Inc., *Toronto*
Prentice-Hall Hispanoamericana, S.A., *Mexico*
Prentice-Hall of India Private Limited, *New Delhi*
Prentice-Hall of Japan, Inc., *Tokyo*
Simon & Schuster Asia Pte. Ltd., *Singapore*
Editora Prentice-Hall do Brasil, Ltda., *Rio de Janeiro*

Contents

Preface

The goal for revising the REGENTS/PRENTICE HALL MEDICAL ASSISTANT KIT was to update and improve the only textbook series written for students of Medical Assisting that integrates the study of anatomy and physiology with diagnosis and treatment of disease. To achieve this goal, we solicited the advice of long-time users of the kit. Their comments resulted in many fundamental changes in the series, including simplification of concepts and procedures; addition of up-to-date information; an emphasis on quality control in all aspects of the physician's office laboratory, and enhanced study aids.

SIMPLIFICATION AND UP-TO-DATE INFORMATION

- Each book emphasizes infection-control consciousness throughout, reflecting the latest OSHA regulations.
- Anatomy and physiology titles have been simplified to reflect the very practical approach many instructors take.
- Diagnoses and treatments of disease have been up-dated for each body system.
- A thoroughly revised BIO-ORGANIZATION launches the anatomy and physiology series with a simplified introduction to the structure and function of the body and a solid foundation for the study of human disease.
- LABORATORY PROCESSES FOR MEDICAL ASSISTING is revised with more than 60% new material, including performance-based procedures checklists for easy instructor evaluation and the latest requirements of the Clinical Laboratory Improvement Act (CLIA).
- CLINICAL PROCESSES FOR MEDICAL ASSISTING now emphasizes only clinical procedures in the POL, leaving administrative issues to other more specific courses.

EMPHASIS ON QUALITY CONTROL

As federal, state, and local regulations become more specific, it is clear that the physicians' major challenge is to provide not only the highest level of quality care and treatment for the patient, but also to document his or her commitment to that quality for the interest of the government. Medical assistants most often execute and police the quality control procedures within the medical office. The new laboratory books emphasize this need for quality control documentation.

The popular "Sources of Error" within the laboratory and clinical procedures checklists have been scrutinized and amplified.

ENHANCED STUDY AIDS

- Knowledge Objectives are grouped by chapter and by section.
- Pronunciations of medical terms are provided the first time a word is used. New terms appear in bold type and are defined in an extensive, updated glossary.
- STOP AND REVIEW sections reflect Knowledge Objectives by section or by chapter.
- Over 60 new or revised illustrations and tables complement the text.
- All illustrations and tables are now precisely referenced in the text.
- Contemporary information in "boxes" add interest and topical information to entice the student.
- Redesigned books emphasize organization and easy reading.
- Two new simplified four-color inserts are: A blood cell chart showing normal and abnormal blood cells; and twelve pages of body systems illustrations to accompany the BIO-ORGANIZATION introduction.
- CLINICAL PROCESSING FOR MEDICAL ASSISTING includes procedures checklists similar to LABORATORY PROCESSES FOR MEDICAL ASSISTING to facilitate instructor evaluation.
- The Laboratory books contain both Knowledge Objectives and Terminal Performance Objectives

PREVIOUS BENEFITS RETAINED

The same strengths and benefits that instructors valued in the past have been retained or expanded:
- The flexible, modular format can be adapted to various program lengths or different sequences of coverage for laboratory, clinical, and anatomy and physiology topics.
- The kit is written in a style specifically appropriate to the medical assisting student.
- The textbook/workbook style enhances student learning. The material remains in small, manageable segments.

- The kit takes an integrated approach to structure, function, and disease of the human body.
- Each body system or medical specialty is followed by its clinical counterpart of disease, diagnosis, and treatment.
- A thorough review of disorders and diseases is classified by type in BIO-ORGANIZATION, and by system throughout the subsequent ten-book series on anatomy and physiology.
- The kit features an emphasis on quality control in LABORATORY PROCESSES FOR MEDICAL ASSISTING and CLINICAL PROCESSES FOR MEDICAL ASSISTING.
- No prior knowledge of biology or chemistry is assumed.

ACKNOWLEDGMENTS

The revision of the Medical Assistant Kit represents the cooperative efforts of many people. Foremost among contributors is Debra Grieneisen, M.T., C.M.A., who served as advisor for the series and in-depth reviser for LABORATORY PROCESSES FOR MEDICAL ASSISTING. Debra has taught medical assisting at Harrisburg Area Community College and Central Pennsylvania Business School. Her commitment to perfection guided this work.

We express gratitude to several medical writers who contributed to these books. They are: Karen Garloff, R.N.; Bruce Goldfarb; Steve Hulse; Ann Moy; and Joy Nixon, R.N.

Cindy Jennings of BMR managed the editorial efforts in this revision. Helping her were Nancy Priff and Rick Stull, as well as Jacqueline Flynn and Greg Flynn.

We particularly want to thank the reviewers whose advice, recommendations and collective knowledge helped form these books. Their primary concern for their students' best interest, the subject matter, and its accuracy are reflected here. One aspect all agreed upon is the importance of accurate, clear illustrations that are integrated and referenced throughout the text. Our reviewers were:

Joanne Bakel
Milton S. Hershey Medical
Center, Hershey, PA

Linda Barrer
Lansdale Business School
Lansdale, PA

Judy Bettinger
Private Medical Practice,
Camp Hill, PA

C. Michael Cronin
California College of Health
Sciences, National City, CA

Martha Faison
Private Medical Practice,
Camp Hill, PA

Irene Figliolina
Berdan Institute, Totowa, NJ

Kathleen Hess
Antonelli Medical & Professional
Institute, Pottstown, PA

Carol Kish
Harrisburg Hospital, Harrisburg, PA

Peter Kish
Harrisburg Area Community College, Harrisburg, PA

Tibby Loveman
Gadsden Business College, Gadsden, AL

Scott McKenzie
Commonwealth College, Virginia Beach, VA

Pat Morelli
Medical Careers Training Center, Ft. Collins, CO

Rhonda O'Grady
The Laboratory Arts Institute, Scarborough, Ontario

Sheila Ritchey
Harrisburg Hospital, Harrisburg, PA

Sandy Rishell
Private Medical Practice, Harrisburg, PA

Janet Sesser
The Bryman School, Phoenix, AZ

Shirley Seekford
Antonelli Medical & Professional Institute, Pottstown, PA

Robert Sheperd
Kee Business College, Norfolk VA

Laura Silva
The Sawyer School, Pawtucket, RI

Pamela Smith
Private Medical Practice, Harrisburg, PA

Bruce Sundrud
Harrisburg Area Community College, Harrisburg, PA

Ann Sugarman
Berdan Institute, Totowa, NJ

Dan Tallman
Northern State University, Aberdeen, SD

Jackie Trentacosta
Galen College, Fresno, CA

Fred Ann Tull
Southern Technical College, Little Rock, AR

Deborah Wood
Concorde Career Institute, Lauderdale Lakes, FL

Finally, we thank those who gave detailed feedback on our questionnaires that helped configure the kit in its present form:

Theresa Bowser
Southern Ohio College, Columbus, OH

Elaine Chamberlin
Pontiac Business Institute, Oxford, MI

Thelma Clavon
Rutledge College, Columbia, SC

Leslie Fiore
Kentucky College of Business, Florence, KY

Diane Franks
National Career College, Tuscaloosa, AL

Tony Gabriel
Watterson College, Pasadena, CA

Karen Greer
Sawyer College, Merrillville, IN

Joyce Hill
Lansdale School of Business, North Wales, PA

Roxanne Holt
Excel College of Medical Arts and
Business, Madison, TN

Annette Jordan
Phillips Business College, Lynchburg,
VA

Martha Juenke
American Medical Training
Institute, Miami, FL

Richard Krafcik
Sawyer College,
Cleveland Heights, OH

Akeeboh Moore
CareerCom College of Business, Oakland, CA

Basil Punsalan
Commonwealth College,
Norfolk, VA

Alta Belle Roberts
Metro Business College, Rolla, MO

Sharon Adams Sasser
Sawyer College, Merrillville, IN

Joyce Shuey
Academy of Medical Arts and
Business, Harrisburg, PA

Mary Ellen Stevenback
Lansdale School of Business,
Harleysville, PA

Jinny Taylor
Academy of Medical Arts and
Business, Harrisburg, PA

Edith Watts
Watterson College, Oxnard, CA

USING THE REVISED MEDICAL ASSISTANT KIT

The ten anatomy and physiology books form the basis for a one-, two-, or three-term introduction to body structure and function and human disease. Each book stands alone and may be used in the most appropriate sequence for your program.

LABORATORY PROCESSES FOR MEDICAL ASSISTING and CLINICAL PROCESSES FOR MEDICAL ASSISTING can supplement the anatomy and physiology books as lab sections or they can be offered as separate courses.

We hope instructors and students alike will find a refreshing clarity and precision in this new edition of the REGENTS PRENTICE HALL MEDICAL ASSISTANT KIT. We look forward to your comments.

Mark Hartman
Editor, Health Professions

The Language of Medicine

As you study this book, you will find that both Latin and Greek words and word parts are used to name organs, diseases and medical procedures. In the study of neurology, we once again have some new word parts. A few examples are:

neur(o)- nerves	(Greek)	*syn-* union, association	(Greek)
ot(o)- ear	(Greek)	*ophthalm(o)-* eye	(Greek)

Use your dictionary when you encounter a word you do not know. The names of many specific nerves are borrowed from words naming sections of the spinal column. These are described in another book in this series, *Orthopedics*. This is a further example of the linkages found in the study of medicine.

Besides using word parts, many words found in neurology are taken directly from other languages. The word will have two meanings—one with a medical meaning and one having nothing to do with neurology. The word creates a picture of the medical characteristic or effect. Some examples of this word usage are:

pons = bridge
cauda equina = horse's tail
astrocytes from the Greek *astron* = star
dendrite from the Greek word for tree

Check the glossary or a dictionary for the neurological meaning of these words.

As you continue your medical training, watch for words that can give you a picture of their meaning. They will help you understand the characteristics and concepts. They will also make it easier for you to relate what you have learned about the various body systems.

The nervous system is one of the most complex systems in the body, and scientists still do not completely understand the details of how it works. If you learn all the information in this book, you will know only a small fraction of what experts in the neurology know.

As you study this material, keep in mind that this is only an introduction to the nervous system. There are many new terms and relationships to learn, and these may be difficult at first. Be prepared to read this material several times in order to gain a good understanding of it. At some points in your study, it may be helpful to review the books in this series on endocrinology and orthopedics to help clarify some of the relationships discussed here.

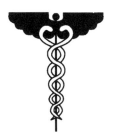

Knowledge Objectives

After completing this chapter, you should be able to:

- describe and name the parts of the central and peripheral nervous systems
- describe the structure and function of the different types of neurons
- explain the structure and purpose of the different types of neuroglia
- describe how nerve impulses function
- explain the function of a synapse
- describe the role of the reflex arc and give some examples
- name and describe the parts and functions of the spinal cord
- name and describe the spinal nerves
- describe the structure and function of the sections of the brain
- list and describe the function and location of the cranial nerves
- describe the structure and function of the brain stem
- describe the structure and function of the cerebellum
- describe the structure, function and parts of the diencephalon
- describe the structure and function of the peripheral nervous system
- describe the functions of the sympathetic and parasympathetic nervous systems

Anatomy of the Nervous System

INTRODUCTION

The nervous system is the major system of communication in the body (see Figure 1). It works closely with the endocrine system (the glands) and the musculoskeletal system. The nervous system controls and organizes activities in the body, both conscious (voluntary) and autonomic (involuntary) functions.

The nervous system also monitors changes within the body, such as blood pressure and blood oxygen, as well as external conditions, such as temperature and other environmental factors. It interprets these changes and adjusts body functions so that a constant internal state or **homeostasis (HOH-mee-oh-STAY-sis)** is maintained.

The nervous system has two major divisions: the **central nervous system (CNS)**, which includes the brain and spinal cord; and the **peripheral nervous system (PNS)**, which includes the nerves that connect the CNS with the body (see Figure 1).

The **autonomic (AW-toh-NOM-ick)** nervous system, which is part of the PNS, organizes and controls those bodily functions over which we normally have no conscious control, and it operates through nerve pathways separate from those over which we have voluntary control.

Neurons (NYOO-ronz), or nerve cells, that carry sensory impulses into the CNS are called **afferent (AF-er-ent)** neurons. Neurons that carry motor impulses from the CNS to the rest of the body are called **efferent (EF-er-ent)** neurons.

These efferent (motor) neurons that carry voluntary messages to skeletal muscles are part of the **somatic (soh-MAT-ick) nervous system**, which stimulates activities such as walking, chewing, or smiling. Those that carry unconscious, involuntary messages to smooth muscles, heart muscle, and glands are part of the autonomic nervous system, which controls digestion, heart activity, and glandular secretions. The CNS controls and integrates all such activities.

The afferent (sensory) neurons, which carry signals to the brain, provide the information necessary for it to make decisions. Should one laugh or cry? Should blood pressure be raised or lowered? Should more blood be distributed to the digestive system or to the muscles? What hormonal messages are needed to avoid an acid-base imbalance in the body? These questions are answered by the brain and spinal cord based on the input provided by the afferent neurons.

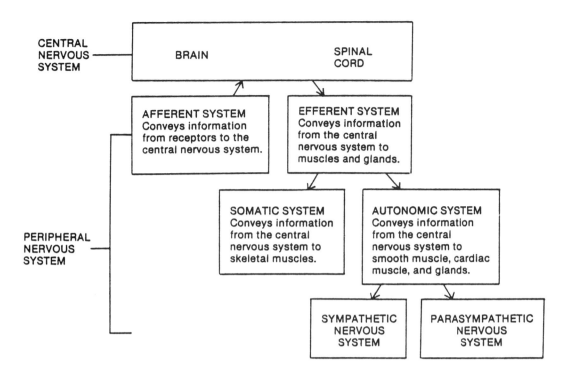

Figure 1: Interaction of the nervous system.

The Cells of the Nervous System

There are two main kinds of cells in the nervous system: neurons and **neuroglia (nyoo-ROG-lee-ah)**. Neurons carry nerve impulses to, from, and within the CNS. They are the working cells of the nervous system. Neuroglia provide the support functions of the system. In a way, they are like the security and maintenance staffs of a big business. There are far more neuroglia than neurons in the nervous system. Most neuroglia are found within the CNS.

Neurons

There are several different types of neurons, but each one has a **cell body** that holds the nucleus of the cell and **processes** or projections that extend out from the cell body. The cell body has a nucleus, a Golgi apparatus **(GOL-jee AP-ah-RAY-tus)** and other typical cell parts. However, a mature nerve cell does not have a centriole, so it cannot reproduce itself. The cytoplasm of the cell extends into

the cell projections, which are called **axons (ACK-sonz)** and **dendrites (DEN-dryts)** (see Figure 2).

The axons and dendrites vary in length from a fraction of an inch to several feet. The nerve cell body must be in a protected place—in the brain, the spinal cord, or a **ganglion (GANG-glee-on)**, which is a nerve center outside the CNS. The dendrites and axons extend from the nerve cell body and carry nerve impulses. Dendrites pick up stimuli and carry them to the cell body. Axons carry impulses to other neurons or to body tissues.

Each neuron has one or more dendrites. These projections have many thread-like branches that look like tree branches. The name dendrite comes from the Greek word for tree. Their tips are called **receptors (ree-SEP-torz)** because they receive stimuli.

Each neuron has a single axon, which may have several branches. An axon may be less than 2 cm long or up to 1 meter long depending on the location of the cell body and the

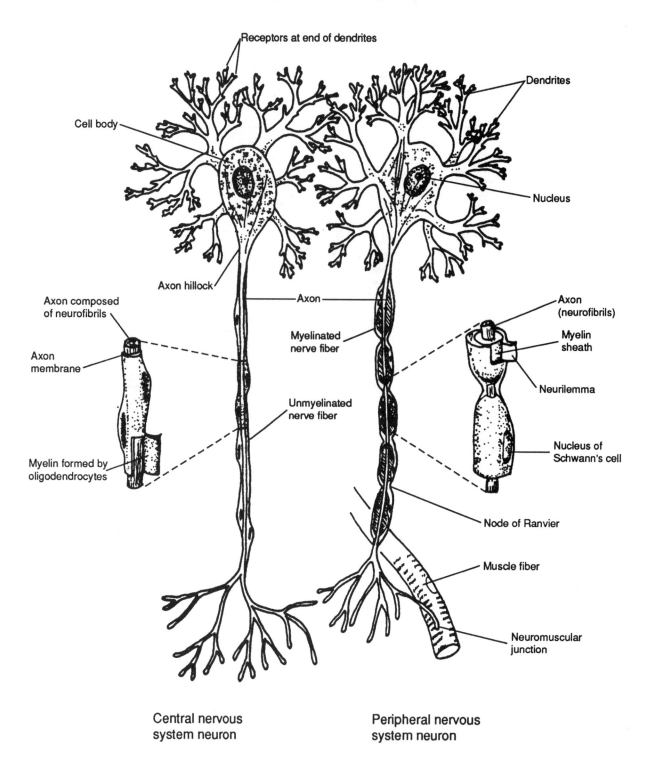

Figure 2: Typical nervous system neurons.

area the neuron is designed to stimulate. For example, if a cell body is in a ganglion near the spinal cord and the neuron stimulates the muscles of the foot, the axon will be a long one. But a neuron in the brain that stimulates a muscle that moves an eyelid will have a short axon. The diameter of axons also varies from about 1μ to 20μ (μ is the symbol for micron, which equals 1/1000 of an inch.) In general, the larger the diameter of the axon, the faster nerve impulses travel along it. The speed of a nerve impulse varies from 18 inches/sec in small, unmyelinated nerves to 100 feet/sec in large, myelinated (**MYE-eh-lih-NAYT-ed**) fibers.

Each axon is attached to its nerve cell body at a site called an **axon hillock**. Some axons are myelinated or wrapped in a layer of lipids and proteins called a **myelin (MYE-eh-lin) sheath**, which is created by other specialized cells. This sheath is not continuous but is interrupted at various intervals by gaps called **neurofibril (NYOO-roh-FIH-bril) nodes** or **nodes of Ranvier (rahn-vee-AY)**.

In the PNS this myelin sheath is formed by **Schwann's (SHVONZ) cells** and is called a **neurilemma (NYOO-rih-LEM-mah)**. It assists the axon in regeneration if severed. A myelin sheath on axons in the brain and spinal cord is formed by **oligodendrocytes (OL-ih-goh-DEN-droh-syts)** and does not form a neurilemma that is capable of allowing regeneration; therefore, damage to neurons in the brain or spinal cord is not reversible. Sometimes, nearby neurons in the system can take over the function of damaged cells, but usually such damage is permanent.

Axons are sometimes referred to as **nerve fibers**. They are grouped together in bundles known as **nerve tracts** in the CNS and simply as **nerves** in the PNS. Bundles of myelinated fibers are also called **white matter** because the myelin gives them a whitish color. Neuron cell bodies grouped together in the CNS and the unmyelinated fibers that go with them have a grayish color and are called **gray matter**. These two kinds of nerve tissue constitute the nervous system.

The gray color of the external surface of the brain is caused by the presence of neurons clustered about the brain's surface (cortex). Cutting into the brain will reveal white matter, indicating the presence of myelinated nerve tracts. An examination of the spinal cord shows white matter (nerve tracts) on the exterior surface and gray matter (neurons) on the interior.

Neuron Types

Neurons can be divided into subgroups according to either their structure or their function. Structurally, there are multipolar, bipolar, and unipolar neurons. The difference is mainly in the number of dendrites and how they relate to the cell body and the axon.

- **Multipolar neurons** have a single axon and several dendrites. Most of them are found in the CNS and function as motor neurons.

- **Bipolar neurons** have one dendrite and one axon. They are the least numerous type and are found in special sense organs such as the eyes and ears.

- **Unipolar neurons** have only one process extending from the cell body, which divides into two processes, an axon and a dendrite. Typically, these are sensory neurons, with their cell bodies often found clustered in enlargements called ganglia.

Functionally, neurons can also be divided into three different subgroups: sensory or afferent neurons; motor or efferent neurons; and interneurons, or connecting neurons.

- **Sensory neurons** (afferent neurons) carry impulses from the rest of the body to the CNS. They detect changes inside and outside the body and convey that information to the CNS.

- **Motor neurons** (efferent neurons) transmit impulses from the CNS to the muscles and glands. When a decision is made, the motor neurons tell the body to carry it out.

- **Interneurons** (central or connecting neurons) form a bridge between sensory neurons and motor neurons. All of them are located in the brain and spinal cord.

To summarize, neurons are the working cells in the nervous system. They are the most varied cells in the body, with extreme variations in size, shape, and general appearance. They are organized into bundles, with their cell bodies grouped together in protected locations in the brain, spinal cord, and ganglia. The processes of the peripheral nerves extend into the rest of the body, but the neurons of the CNS are contained completely within that system. The neuroglia provide the structures that surround, protect, and support the neurons.

Neuroglia

These supportive cells in the CNS have five different specialized types.

Astrocytes (AS-troh-syts).   These are star-shaped cells, and their name comes from *astron*, the Greek word for star. They have a central cell body and many processes or projections. They are found mainly in the brain and spinal cord between the neurons and the blood vessels that supply the system with nourishment. Astrocytes probably have a role in controlling the blood supply to the CNS.

Oligodendrocytes.   These cells are smaller and have fewer processes than astrocytes. They surround nerve cell bodies and their extensions and hold them together in bundles or tracts. They also provide a covering (the myelin sheath) for neurons in the central nervous system.

Microglia (mye-KROG-lee-ah).   These are small cells that are normally stationary. When brain tissue is inflamed or damaged, however, microglia enlarge and begin to move. They remove debris and infection in the brain through a process of engulfing and digesting called **phagocytosis (FAG-oh-sye-TOH-sis).**

Ependymal (eh-PEN-dih-mal) *cells.* These are similar to epithelial cells in other parts of the body. They form the inner lining of the cavities in the brain—called **ventricles (VEN-trih-kulz)**—and of the central canal in the spinal cord.

Schwann's cells.   These are tiny, flat cells that wrap around the nerve fibers of many neurons. They form a covering known as the neurilemma or the **sheath of Schwann**. In the PNS, the myelin sheath is made from the membranes of Schwann cells.

In general, neuroglia form the connective tissue of the nervous system. But unlike other connective tissues in the body, they are soft and jelly-like, not fibrous or elastic.

STOP AND REVIEW

Short answers

1. Name the two other systems with which the nervous system works closely.

    a. _____

    b. _____

2. Name two major divisions of the nervous system.

    a. _____

    b. _____

3. Name the two main kinds of cells in the nervous system.

   a. _____

   b. _____

4. Name the five types of neuroglia.

   a. _____

   b. _____

   c. _____

   d. _____

   e. _____

5. Define and describe the function of a dendrite.

   _____

   _____

6. Define and describe the function of an axon.

   _____

   _____

7. What are the main structural differences among unipolar, bipolar, and multipolar neurons? _____

   _____

8. Name the three types of neurons in terms of their function.

   a. _____

   b. _____

   c. _____

9. Name the most common type of cell found in nerve tissue. _____

NERVE CELL PHYSIOLOGY

Neurons function by carrying or conducting nerve impulses or messages from one part of the body to another. To do this, neurons must have two properties: **excitability (eck-SYT-ah-BIL-ih-tee)** and **conductivity (KON-duck-TIV-ih-tee)**. Excitability is the ability to be affected by a stimulus, and conductivity is the ability to transmit that stimulus as a nerve impulse.

Nerve impulses are the fastest method of communication within the body. Each one is rapidly sent and short-lived. (The endocrine system and its hormones are controlled by nerve impulses and cause slower but longer-lasting modifications of body functions.) For sustained actions, a series of impulses along a set of related but separate neurons is required.

Nerve Impulses

Nerve impulses travel along the axons of individual neurons in a complex set of electrical and chemical reactions. Before this can happen, the nerve must be at rest and it must receive a stimulus. The stimulus can occur at any point along the axon, but most often it begins at the receptors at the end of the dendrites, then moves to the axon hillock and from there along the length of the axon.

To start a nerve impulse, a stimulus must be strong enough to begin the process and also appropriate to the particular neuron. Neurons are highly specialized in their function. For example, sound waves stimulate neurons that are part of the auditory nerve, and heat stimulates temperature receptors on the skin. But ordinarily heat cannot initiate an impulse in an auditory nerve, and temperature receptors are not stimulated by sound waves.

When a stimulus does initiate a nerve impulse, it is known as **adequate stimulus**. Once an impulse begins, it travels the whole length of the axon at a set strength and speed. If the stimulus is not adequate, no impulse occurs. This is known as the *all or nothing response*.

The impulse itself works as follows (see Figure 3). First the nerve must be at rest. When it is at rest, a nerve contains more negatively charged ions than positively charged ions in its cytoplasm. (An ion is an atom that has an unequal number of protons [positive charges] or electrons [negative charges].) Positively charged potassium is present inside the cells but not in a large enough proportion to dominate the cytoplasm. Outside the nerve cell membrane, the environment has more positively charged ions, many of them sodium ions. The membrane is relatively impermeable to

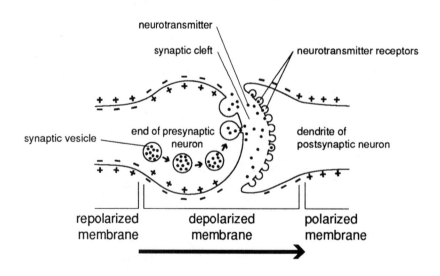

Figure 3: Impulse transmission at synapse.

these particles, so a balance is maintained—a positive charge outside the membrane and a negative charge inside the cell. This situation is known as a **resting potential**. The cell is at rest, but it is ready to respond to an adequate stimulus, so it has a potential for action.

When an adequate stimulus occurs, the cell membrane becomes permeable to sodium at the point of stimulation. At that point, sodium rushes into the cell. This changes the electrical balance in the affected section of the cell. It becomes more positive than negative inside, and more negative than positive outside. This reversal is known as **depolarization (dee-POH-lar-ih-ZAY-shun)**.

When a portion of a nerve cell membrane depolarizes, it causes the cell membrane next to that portion to also become permeable to sodium and therefore it also depolarizes. This causes depolarization to move along the neuron in an advancing wave.

As the depolarization wave passes, the membrane immediately becomes impermeable to sodium but temporarily permeable to potassium, which then rushes outside the cell to restore the original resting potential. Thus, a nerve impulse can be described as a depolarization wave followed by a repolarization wave.

After a nerve impulse passes, the sodium and potassium are restored to their original locations through a mechanism known as the **sodium-potassium pump**, found in the neuron's cell membrane.

Local anesthetics such as procaine prevent the nerve membrane from becoming permeable to sodium. This prevents nerve impulses along a pain pathway from proceeding beyond the point of anesthesia.

The progress of a stimulus along the neuron is called an **action potential**. The action potential moves along the neuron until it reaches the other end of the axon. Then it must move either to the muscle or gland to which it is carrying the impulse (for a motor neuron) or to the next nerve (for a sensory neuron or an interneuron).

In myelinated nerve fibers, the myelin sheath serves as an insulator. It prevents both sodium and potassium from moving across the cell membrane. However, the myelin sheath is not continuous; it is interrupted at intervals along the length of the axon. These interruptors are called neurofibril nodes (nodes of Ranvier). When a nerve impulse travels along a myelinated axon, the impulse jumps from node to node instead of moving smoothly along the axon membrane. This form of impulse conduction is called **saltatory conduction**. This type of conduction allows the impulse to travel five to seven times faster than with continuous conduction.

Synapse

A **synapse (SIN-aps)** is the junction between two neurons. When a nerve impulse reaches the end of a **presynaptic (PREE-sih-NAP-tick) neuron**, it causes the nerve ending to release a substance called a **neurotransmitter (NYOO-roh-TRANS-mit-er)**, which will affect the resting potential of the **postsynaptic (POST-sih-NAP-tick) neuron** (see Figure 3).

These neurotransmitters are contained in the nerve endings in tiny sacs called **vesicles (VES-ih-kulz)**. A nerve impulse will cause some of these vesicles to release their neurotransmitters, which will then diffuse across the narrow gap between the two neurons called the **synaptic cleft (sih-NAP-tick CLEFT)** and affect the postsynaptic neuron.

If the neurotransmitter causes the postsynaptic neuron to increase it polarity (which will make it less likely to depolarize), it is an in-hibitory, **(in-HIB-ih-TOR-ee)** neurotransmitter. Examples of inhibitory neurotransmitters include **gamma-aminobutyric acid (GAM-mah ah-MEE-noh-BYOO-tih-rick AS-id) (GABA)**, **glycine (GLYE-seen)**, and **dopamine (DOH-pah-meen)**.

If the neurotransmitter causes the postsynaptic neuron to decrease its polarity (bringing it closer to depolarization), it is an excitatory **(eck-SYE-tah-TOH-ree)** neurotransmitter. Examples of excitatory neurotransmitters include **acetylcholine (AS-eh-til-KOH-leen) (ACh)**, **norepinephrine (NOR-ep-ih-NEF-rin)**, **serotonin (SER-oh-TOH-nin)**, and **histamine (HIS-tah-meen)**. Caffeine lowers the postsynaptic nerve's threshold, making it possible for a lesser amount of excitatory neurotransmitter to cause it to depolarize. That is why caffeine acts as a nerve stimulant.

Because only presynaptic nerve endings contain neurotransmitters, a synapse can only carry messages in one direction.

The main advantage of synapses in the nervous system is that they allow decision-making to take place. This is because several presynaptic neurons may connect with a particular postsynaptic neuron. For example, although removing a splinter might cause a reflex (pulling away of the hand), higher nerve centers (following the admonishment to "hold still!") can deliver sufficient inhibitory neurotransmitters at the reflex synapse to hold the hand still and override the reflex.

Synapses allow control over which sensory impulses will be carried on to higher nerve centers and which motor impulses will be carried back to the body, thus providing remarkable order and regulation over the entire nervous system.

The Reflex Arc

In general, the nervous system functions through a series of events known as the **reflex arc**. A reflex arc is the shortest route an impulse can take from a receptor to an **effector (ef-FECK-tor)**, a muscle or gland that performs a specific action when stimulated. Such an arc can involve a few nerve fibers or many, and it can be simple or complex. The simplest reflexes require only two neurons—one receptor and one effector. The receptor receives a stimulus and transmits it to the CNS through a sensory neuron. There it crosses a synapse to a motor neuron, which sends an appropriate message to the affected part of the body. This type of reflex is called a **monosynaptic reflex**. A classic example is the patellar reflex: a sharp blow to the kneecap (patella) tendon causes an immediate extension of the lower leg (see Figure 4). (If the patellar reflex does not occur

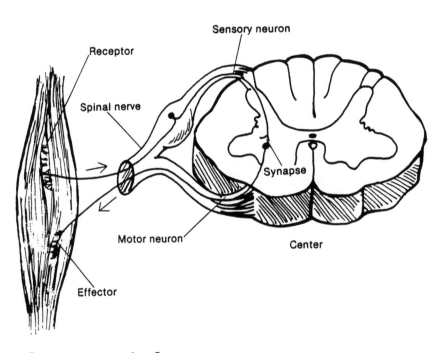

Figure 4: The patellar reflex, a monosynaptic reflex.

during testing, the patient might have a problem in the thigh muscle, femoral nerve, or spinal cord.) The patellar reflex is also an example of the **stretch reflex**, which is the reflex contraction of a muscle in response to passive stretching.

In more complex reflex arcs, the stimulus goes first from the receptor, through the sensory neuron to an interneuron which interprets the message and "instructs" a third neuron to respond. Usually a set of related reflexes occurs in more than one set of neurons at the same time.

The nervous system consists of bundles or tracts of individual neurons. These resemble a sophisticated telephone cable. They convey many stimuli from the body to the brain and spinal cord. Those stimuli are sorted and interpreted in the CNS, where the interneurons are located. Then a response is directed out again to the appropriate site. The CNS has two separate but related structures—the spinal cord and the brain. These will each be discussed in the next two sections of this chapter.

STOP AND REVIEW

Fill in the blanks

1. The ability to be affected by a stimulus is called _____

2. The ability to transmit a stimulus as a nerve impulse is called _____

3. A nerve at rest contains more _____ (positive/negative) ions than _____ (positive/negative) ions in its cytoplasm.

4. Repolarization occurs when the cell acquires a more _____ (positive/negative) charge on the inside and a more_____ (positive/negative) charge on the outside.

5. The shortest route a nerve impulse can take from a receptor to an effector is called the _____

Short answers

6. Define the term "adequate stimulus." _____

   _____

7. How do nerve impulses travel across the synapse? _____

   _____

True or False

8. Neurotransmitter chemical substances that make the neuron more excitable are:

   a. ____ acetylcholine

   b. ____ dopamine

   c. ____ glycine

   d. ____ histamine

   e. ____ serotonin

   f. ____ gamma-aminobutyric acid

ANATOMY OF THE SPINAL CORD

The spinal cord is a long, thin, tubular structure consisting of a combination of gray matter inside and white matter outside. In an adult, the spinal cord measures about 45 cm. It includes myelinated and unmyelinated neurons, as well as neuron cell bodies, all surrounded and supported by neuroglial cells. This organ begins at the base of the brain, at the **medulla oblongata (Meh-DUL-ah OB-long-GAH-tah)**, and extends to the **second lumbar vertebra (LUM-ber VER-teh-brah)** in adults. It fits neatly into the circular opening in the center of the vertebral arch, so it is protected by the bony spine. The spinal nerves project out from the cord on both sides to form the PNS.

The nerves of the upper and lower extremities project from enlargements at the top and bottom of the spinal cord. The enlargement at the top is the **cervical (SER-vih-kal) enlargement**, and the one at the bottom is the **lumbar enlargement**.

The spinal cord is divided in half lengthwise to form right and left sides (see Figure 5). On the anterior or ventral side, the division is made by a deep groove called the **anterior** or **ventral median fissure (VEN-tral MEE-dee-an FISH-yoor)**. On the posterior or dorsal side is a shallower groove called the **posterior** or **dorsal median sulcus (DOR-sal MEE-dee-an SUL-kus)**. A bridge of gray and white matter joins the two portions in the midsection of the cord. This is called a **commissure (KOM-ih-shyoor)**.

Through the center of the cord runs an open space called the **central canal**. This space, which extends the entire length of the cord, is filled with a fluid known as **cerebrospinal (SER-eh-broh-SPYE-nal) fluid** (CSF). The canal is connected to ventricles (or spaces) in the brain and the subarachnoid space over the brain that also contain this fluid.

The spinal cord tapers to a point at the bottom of its structure. This section is called the **conus medullaris (KOH-nus MED-yoo-LAY-ris)**. A number of nerves originate at the

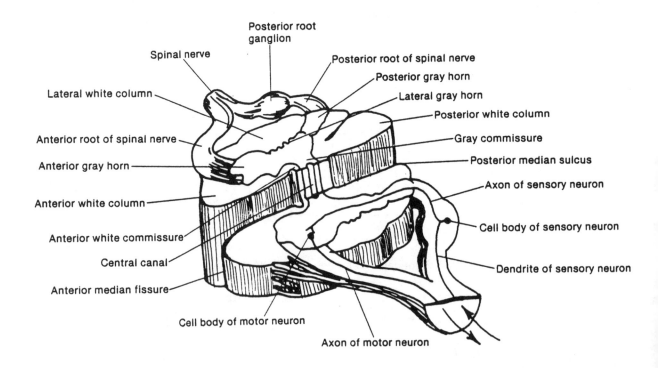

Figure 5: Spinal cord, cross-section.

end of the cord and extend below it within the spinal column to openings in the lumbar vertebrae and the coccyx. These nerve roots are known collectively as the **cauda equina (KAW-dahy eh-kwyne-ah)**; meaning "horse's tail", because they resemble the tail of a horse.

A cross-section of the spinal cord shows an oval structure with a roughly H-shaped area of gray tissue in the center and white tissue around it. It consists of neuron cell bodies and unmyelinated axons. The legs of the "H" of gray matter are called **horns**.

The white matter consists of myelinated nerve fibers or axons bound together in nerve tracts. These are arranged in columns or **funiculi (fyoo-NICK-yoo-lye)**. Each column has **ascending tracts**, which carry nerve impulses from the rest of the body to the brain, and **descending tracts**, which carry impulses in the opposite direction. Ascending tracts are also called **sensory tracts**, because they deliver sensations to the brain. Descending tracts are called **motor tracts**, because they cause motion.

The spinal cord is covered on the outside by three layers of tissue, known collectively as the **meninges (meh-NIN-jeez)**, which also cover the brain. The three layers, starting with the outermost layer, are the **dura mater (DYOO-rah MAY-ter)**, the **arachnoid (ah-RACK-noyd)**, and the **pia mater (PYE-ah MAY-ter)**. Between the dura mater and the vertebrae is a space known as the **extradural (ECKS-trah-DYOO-ral)** space; it is filled with blood vessels and connective tissue. The vertebral ligaments, which are attached to the meninges, are within this space and hold the cord in place. There is a very narrow space between the dura mater and the arachnoid layer and a larger space between the arachnoid and the pia mater called the **subarachnoid (SUB-ah-**

RACK-noyd) space. The subarachnoid space is filled with cerebrospinal fluid. The pia mater is a delicate membrane filled with blood vessels. It is very close to the cord (almost part of it) and supplies the cells within the cord with oxygen and nutrients.

The spinal cord has two main functions. One is to convey information to and from the brain. The other is to serve as a reflex center. Remember that nerve cell bodies are found in the spinal cord, brain, and ganglia. For a reflex arc to be completed, a message must go to one of these central locations via a sensory nerve and be relayed to a motor nerve to complete the reflex. The spinal cord provides the shortest route for such messages. Complex actions take more time and may have to be processed by the brain before a response to a stimulus is selected.

In some reflexes, the neurons are on one side of the spinal cord. This is known as an **ipsilateral (IP-sih-LAT-er-al) reflex**. In others, the neurons cross from one side to the other. This is a **contralateral (KON-trah**

THERAPEUTIC USES OF THE SUBARACHNOID SPACE

During a lumbar puncture, a needle is placed into the subarachnoid space around the spinal cord and cerebrospinal fluid is withdrawn for analysis. To avoid damage to the cord itself, the puncture is made between the third and fourth lumbar vertebrae. The conus medullaris is located at the approximate level of the second lumbar vertebra. Anesthesia can be administered through a needle placed in the same location as a lumbar puncture. If the anesthetic is injected above the dura mater, it is called an epidural and may require several minutes to take effect. If the anesthetic is injected below the dura mater, it is called a spinal and anesthesia is accomplished almost immediately. The change in pressure in the cerebrospinal fluid might unfortunately cause what is termed a "spinal" headache.

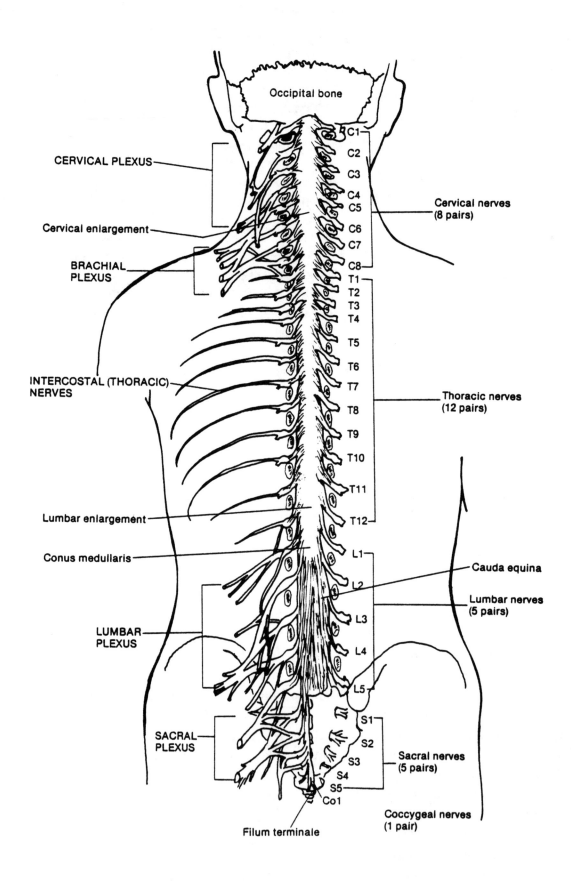

Occipital bone

CERVICAL PLEXUS

Cervical enlargement

BRACHIAL PLEXUS

INTERCOSTAL (THORACIC) NERVES

Lumbar enlargement

Conus medullaris

LUMBAR PLEXUS

SACRAL PLEXUS

Filum terminale

C1
C2
C3
C4
C5
C6
C7
C8

T1
T2
T3
T4
T5
T6
T7
T8
T9
T10
T11
T12

L1
L2
L3
L4
L5

S1
S2
S3
S4
S5
Co1

Cervical nerves (8 pairs)

Thoracic nerves (12 pairs)

Cauda equina

Lumbar nerves (5 pairs)

Sacral nerves (5 pairs)

Coccygeal nerves (1 pair)

Figure 6: Spinal cord and nerves, posterior view.

LAT-er-al) reflex.

The Spinal Nerves

There are 31 pairs of spinal nerves. They are named and numbered after the vertebrae in the part of the spine where each nerve emerges (see Figure 6). For example, the first cervical nerve or C-1 is at the top of the spinal column at the level of the first cervical vertebra. There are eight pairs of cervical nerves, 12 pairs of **thoracic (thoh-RAS-ick) nerves**, five pairs of **lumbar nerves**, and five pairs of **sacral (SAY-kral) nerves**. The lumbar and sacral nerves compose the cauda equina. At the very bottom of the cauda equina is the last pair, which stem from the **coccygeal (kock-SIJ-eeal) nerve**.

Each spinal nerve is attached to the spinal cord by two roots—a **dorsal** or **posterior root** and a **ventral** or **anterior root**. The dorsal root contains sensory nerves. It has a swelling on it called a **dorsal root ganglion**, which holds the cell bodies of sensory (afferent) neurons. The ventral root contains motor (efferent) neurons. Their cell bodies are in the ventral horns of the gray matter of the cord, so the ventral root does not include a ganglion.

The spinal nerves are referred to as **mixed nerves** because they contain both sensory and motor neurons. Each spinal nerve, except C-1, provides nerves to a specific area of the skin called a **dermatome (DER-mah-tohm)**. A physician can test the responses in these areas to determine which spinal nerve is diseased or damaged.

Each spinal nerve branches into the **dorsal ramus (RAY-mus)**, (plural: rami) and the **ventral ramus**. In all but the first 11 thoracic nerves (T-1 to T-11), the ventral ramus of each nerve

PLEXUS INJURIES

A nerve plexus can be injured. For example, the solar plexus, located in the center of the abdomen, controls the stomach, liver, and kidneys. A sharp blow to this area can cause extreme pain or even loss of consciousness.

joins with the ventral rami of other neighboring nerves to form networks of smaller nerves called **plexuses (PLECK-sus-es)**. The major plexuses are the **cervical**, **brachial (BRAY-kee-al) lumbar**, and **sacral plexuses**. They are named after the general regions of the body that they serve. From these networks come smaller branches of the nerves, which innervate (or serve) muscles, organs, glands, and so forth. These nerves also are named after the areas or structures they innervate.

The thoracic nerves are also called the **intercostal (IN-ter-KOS-tal) nerves**, after the formal name for the ribs, **costae (KOS-tee)**. They innervate structures within the rib area, and they go directly to their destinations without forming plexuses.

Spinal reflexes are important to the person with an injured spinal cord. Even though messages cannot travel to and from the brain, spinal reflexes allow the bowel and bladder to continue functioning if the level of injury is above the eleventh thoracic vertebra (T-11). Below this level, a lack of spinal reflexes makes it more difficult for the injured person to manage bowel and bladder functions.

Reflexes are important to the able-bodied person as well. For example, reflexes cause us to quickly withdraw from painful stimuli before we consciously sense the pain, often preventing serious injury.

THE BRAIN

The brain is the central switchboard of the nervous system (see Figure 7). It is an incredibly complex organ, and researchers are constantly discovering new information about how it works. There are billions of neurons in the brain and millions of synaptic connections between them. The cranial nerves, which innervate the head and face and associated organs, originate on the underside of the brain (see Figure 8). For the names of the cranial nerves and information about the functions each one controls, see Table 1.

The brain is organized into four main sections (see Figure 7): the **cerebral hemispheres (SER-eh-bral HEM-ih-sfeerz)** or **cerebrum (SER-eh-brum)**, the **cerebellum (SER-eh-BEL-um)**, the **diencephalon (DYE-en-SEF-ah-lon)**, and the **brain stem (BRAYN stem)**. The whole is sometimes called the **encephalon (en-SEF-ah-lon)**. Each part has its own particular role in coordinating and controlling body functions and activities. Before looking at these sections in detail, we will review the protective coverings of the brain, its blood supply, and some other general information about how it is organized.

Like the spinal cord, the brain has a bony covering and a covering of three layers of tissue. The bony protection of the brain is composed of the bones of the skull. The major cranial bones are the **frontal, parietal (pah-RYE-eh-tal), occipital (ock-SIP-ih-tal), temporal (TEM-poh-ral), sphenoid (SFEE-noyd)**, and **ethmoid (ETH-moyd) bones**. They join to form a single rounded box that fits closely around the brain and prevents all but the severest blows from injuring the brain.

The tissue coverings or meninges are continuous with the coverings of the spinal cord (see Figure 9). The dura mater actually has two layers in the section that covers the brain. One adheres to the interior of the skull, and

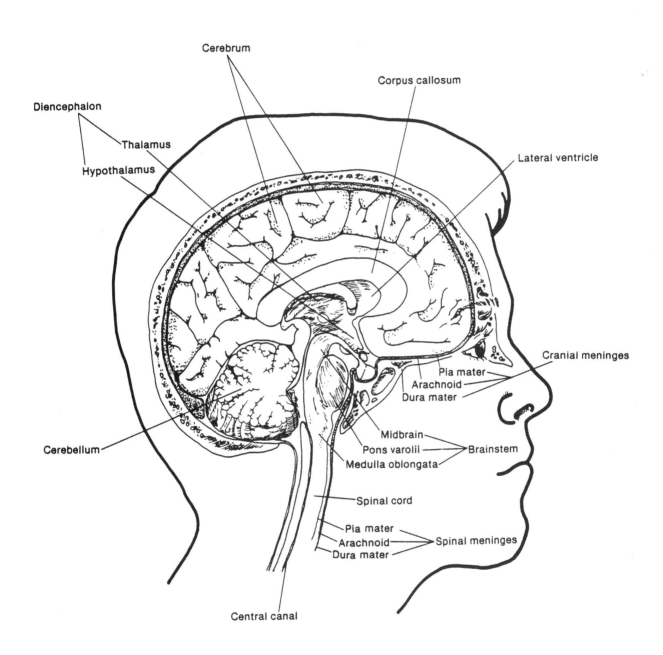

Diencephalon

Thalamus

Hypothalamus

Cerebrum

Corpus callosum

Lateral ventricle

Cranial meninges

Pia mater
Arachnoid
Dura mater

Cerebellum

Midbrain
Pons varolii
Medulla oblongata

Brainstem

Spinal cord

Pia mater
Arachnoid
Dura mater

Spinal meninges

Central canal

Figure 7: The brain.

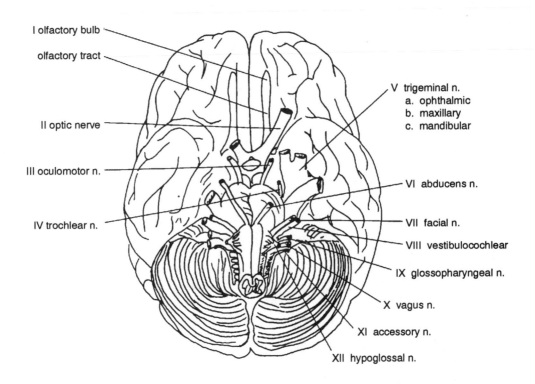

I olfactory bulb
olfactory tract
II optic nerve
III oculomotor n.
IV trochlear n.

V trigeminal n.
  a. ophthalmic
  b. maxillary
  c. mandibular
VI abducens n.
VII facial n.
VIII vestibulocochlear
IX glossopharyngeal n.
X vagus n.
XI accessory n.
XII hypoglossal n.

Figure 8: Base of the brain and the points of origin of the cranial nerves

the other is in contact with its partner except where it follows the contours of a fissure or division in the brain's surface. In those areas, there is a space between the layers of the dura mater, and these spaces are filled with blood. They are called **cranial sinuses** and serve as the venous system for the brain. That is, blood that has delivered its oxygen and nutrients to the cells leaves the brain by way of these sinuses.

As in the spinal cord, the arachnoid membrane is next. It is held above the pia mater and the surface of the brain by a structure of tiny extensions called **trabeculae (trah-BECK-yoo-lee)**. The space thus formed is filled with CSF. Next is the pia mater, which lies close to the surface of the brain and follows every contour of its convoluted surface.

The CSF in the subarachnoid space makes the meninges a fluid-filled cushion as well as a covering. Cerebrospinal fluid is clear, colorless, and watery. It is composed of a combination of interstitial fluid that filters out of the capillaries of the brain and fluid formed by **the choroid (KOH-royd) plexuses**, networks of blood vessels in the ventricles of the brain. The ventricles are open spaces in the central part of the brain that connect to both the subarachnoid space and the central canal of the spinal cord (see Figure 7). The fluid circulates in a regular route through these cavities. It is continuously produced and then absorbed into the bloodstream to maintain a constant amount. It contains water, sodium chloride, potassium, glucose, a small amount of protein, and a few white blood cells.

The CSF supports and protects the brain and spinal cord. It acts as a shock absorber to cushion the CNS from bumps and blows. A blood-CSF fluid barrier prevents some harmful substances, including certain drugs, bacteria, and toxins (poisons), from entering the CSF. Cerebrospinal fluid can be removed from the lower part of the spinal cord and tested to see if the fluid in the brain is normal because the same fluid circulates throughout the CNS.

Table 1: The Cranial Nerves

Name (Sensory/Motor)*	Function	Origin/Destination
I. Olfactory (Ol-FACK-toh-ree) (S)	Sense of smell	Dendrites and cell bodies in nasal mucous membrane to axons in olfactory bulbs and temporal lobe of cerebrum
II. Optic (S)	Vision	Retina to thalamus and posterior lobe of cerebral cortex
III. Oculomotor (OCK-yoo-loh-MOH-tor) (M)	Movement of eyeball and eyelid, regulation of pupil size, accommodation for close vision	Midbrain to eye muscles
IV. Trochlear (TROCK-lee-ar) (M)	Movement of eyeball	Midbrain to eye muscles (superior oblique)
V. Trigeminal (trye-JEM-ih-nal) (S and M)	Ophthalmic branch; maxillary branch; mandibular branch Sensation in head and face; chewing	Face, eyelids, surface of eye, tear glands, nose, scalp, forehead, teeth, jaws, lips, gums to pons; pons to chewing muscles
VI. Abducens (ab-DYOO-senz) (M)	Eye movement	Pons to eye muscles (lateral rectus)
VII. Facial (S and M)	Taste; facial expressions; secretion of tears and saliva	Tongue to medulla; pons-medulla junction to facial muscles, tear and saliva glands
VIII. Vestibulocochlear (ves-TIB-yoo-loh-KOCK-lee-ar) (S)	Cochlear branch; vestibular branch; hearing; balance	Inner ear to pons-medulla junction and midbrain
IX. Glossopharyngeal (GLOS-oh-fah-RIN-jee-al) (S and M)	Taste; swallowing; secretion of saliva	Tongue to medulla; medulla to muscles of pharynx to salivary glands
X. Vagus (VAY-gus) (S and M)	Sensation in larynx, trachea, heart, stomach, and other organs; movement of organs	Organs to medulla; medulla to organ muscles and glands
XI. Spinal accessory (M)	Movement of shoulders and head	Medulla and spinal cord to muscles of shoulders, head, pharynx, and larynx
XII. Hypoglossal (HYE-poh-GLOS-al) (M)	Tongue movement	Medulla to tongue muscles

* Some nerves designated as motor only have some minor sensory functions—they include III, IV, VI, XI, XII.

As noted earlier the veins that carry blood out of the brain are the cranial sinuses. The main arteries that supply the brain with oxygen and nutrients form a circle at the base of the brain called the **circle of Willis**. This structure provides many alternate routes for that essential blood supply to reach the brain. If the nerve tissue does not receive enough oxygen, nerve cells weaken and die. Eventually, if circulation is not restored, the brain ceases to function and death follows. The circle of arteries functions as a safeguard against damage or blockage in any one of these vital arteries. From the circle, three pairs of cerebral arteries carry blood into the interior of the brain.

A mechanism called the **blood-brain barrier** regulates which materials in the bloodstream can enter the brain. Chemical deficiencies or excesses in the brain cause the arteries to either constrict or dilate until the balance is restored. The brain is especially sensitive to the oxygen/carbon dioxide balance (re-

THE IMPORTANCE OF BLOOD FLOW TO THE BRAIN

Maintaining adequate oxygen and blood flow to the brain is critical. Permanent brain damage results within 4 to 6 minutes after cardiac arrest (stoppage of the heart). Biological death (the death of brain cells) occurs within 10 minutes after cardiac arrest.

flected by the acid-base balance) and to the level of glucose it receives. Glucose deficiency in the brain can cause dizziness, convulsions, or unconsciousness.

The brain is also supplied with more than 40 different neurotransmitter chemicals. These chemicals regulate nerve impulses by exciting, inhibiting, or facilitating those impulses as they cross synapses between neurons. Some act as painkillers, and others are hormones or related compounds that govern muscular and glandular responses to nerve impulses (see Table 2).

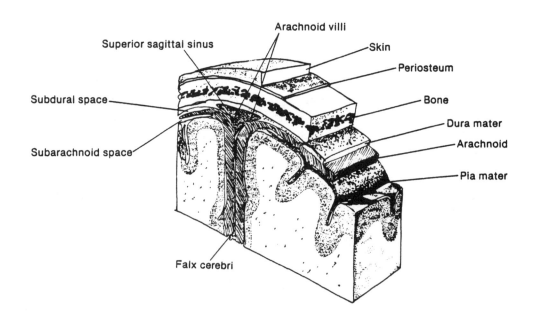

Figure 9: Cranial meninges.

Table 2: Neurotransmitter Chemicals in the Brain

Many chemicals in the brain are known or suspected to be neurotransmitters. The chemical names of some examples are given below. They are divided into groups according to their functions.

- **Excitors**: acetylcholine (ACh), norepinephrine (NE), serotonin (5-HT), **glutamic (gloo-TAH-mick) acid, aspartic (ah-SPAR-tick) acid**, histamine
- **Inhibitors**: gamma-aminobutyric acid (GABA), glycine, dopamine (DA)
- **Painkillers** (inhibitors of pain impulses): **enkephalins (en-KEF--ah-linz), endorphins (en-DOR-finz)**
- Hormones (regulators of physiological responses): **angiotensin (AN-jee-oh-TEN-sin), chole-cystokinin (KOH-lee-SIS-toh-KIN-in), neurotensin (NYOO-roh-TEN-sin) hypothalamic (HYE-poh-thah-LAM-ick) regulators**

For more information on hormones and how they function, see the book on endocrinology in this series.

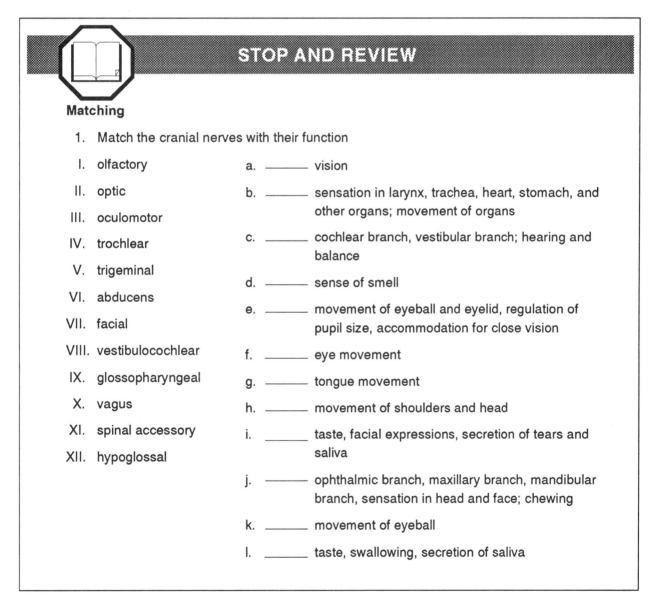

STOP AND REVIEW

Matching

1. Match the cranial nerves with their function

I. olfactory	a. _____ vision
II. optic	b. _____ sensation in larynx, trachea, heart, stomach, and other organs; movement of organs
III. oculomotor	
IV. trochlear	c. _____ cochlear branch, vestibular branch; hearing and balance
V. trigeminal	d. _____ sense of smell
VI. abducens	e. _____ movement of eyeball and eyelid, regulation of pupil size, accommodation for close vision
VII. facial	
VIII. vestibulocochlear	f. _____ eye movement
IX. glossopharyngeal	g. _____ tongue movement
X. vagus	h. _____ movement of shoulders and head
XI. spinal accessory	i. _____ taste, facial expressions, secretion of tears and saliva
XII. hypoglossal	
	j. _____ ophthalmic branch, maxillary branch, mandibular branch, sensation in head and face; chewing
	k. _____ movement of eyeball
	l. _____ taste, swallowing, secretion of saliva

THE PARTS OF THE BRAIN

We will look now at the sections of the brain, beginning with the brain stem and working up to the cerebral hemispheres.

The Brain Stem

The part of the brain that is called the stem looks very much like a stem or a handle when viewed from the side. It has three parts: the medulla oblongata, the **pons (PONZ)** and the **midbrain**.

The lowest part of the brain stem is the medulla oblongata and is a continuation of the spinal cord. It contains tracts of white matter that are the channels of communication between the spinal cord and the brain. Many of these tracts cross from one side of the body to the other in the medulla—these tracts are called the pyramids. The medulla also contains some gray matter called nuclei. These are cell bodies for the last four cranial nerves IX to XII and a number of reflex centers. The centers regulate heart rate, respiratory rate, vasoconstriction, swallowing, coughing, vomiting, sneezing, and hiccupping.

The pons is the middle section of the brain stem. The term literally means "bridge," and the pons does serve as a bridge between the spinal cord and brain and from one part of the brain to another. Cranial nerves VI, VII, VIII, and X originate in the pons. These control areas of the face, hearing and balance, blood pressure, and heart rate. Also, a group of neurons in the base of the pons forms the pneumotaxic center, which helps to regulate breathing.

The **midbrain** is a small section of nerve tissue that connects the pons to the lower portion of the cerebrum. A narrow canal passes through the midbrain that carries cerebrospinal fluid from the third ventricle (in the diencephalon) to the fourth ventricle (in the back of the brain stem, leading to the spinal cord). Cranial nerves III and IV originate in this part of the brain stem.

Centers for visual and auditory reflexes and postural reflexes are also found in the midbrain. Visual reflexes include constriction and dilation of the pupil in response to light. Auditory reflexes involve moving the head to pick up sounds. Postural and righting reflexes are related to staying right side up and keeping the head, eyes, and limbs adjusted to changes in posture.

The Cerebellum

The cerebellum, which means "little brain," is attached to the brain stem below the cerebral hemisphere and behind the brain stem. The outside of it consists of gray matter arranged in narrow folds. Inside is a tree-like arrangement of white matter, which is composed of tracts of myelinated nerve fibers. The cerebellum is attached to the cerebrum and the medulla and spinal cord by bundles of fibers called **peduncles (peh-DUNG-kulz)**.

The cerebellum coordinates muscular movement. When the cerebrum signals for a particular action, such as pushing a button, the cerebellum senses the original position of the body and the changes that occur around joints as the movement takes place. While doing this, it constantly modifies the messages to the muscles involved so that the motion is smooth, coordinated, and skillful. The clumsiness of a person learning a new task soon disappears as the cerebellum is trained. Even such movements as speech are highly coordinated by the cerebellum. During rapid movements such as in running or swinging the arms, the cerebellum helps the brain predict the future position of body parts based on their current location and the speed and direction of movement. Cerebellar damage from injury or disease results in a neurological "loss of limbs"; that is, the person cannot tell where his or her arms or legs are located while in motion.

The Diencephalon

This area of the brain is located under the cerebral hemispheres, where the midbrain joins the brain stem to the rest of the brain. It surrounds the third ventricle of the brain. The diencephalon consists of the **thalamus (THAL-ah-mus)** and the **hypothalamus (HYE-poh-THAL-ah-mus)**. Both of these centers provide linkages between the higher centers of the cerebral hemispheres, where decisions are made, and the body, where those decisions are carried out

The Thalamus. There actually are two thalami, one on each side of the third ventricle. These centers form most of the tissue of the diencephalon and consist of nerve cell bodies or gray matter. Their function is to relay sensations from all parts of the body, except the nose, to the brain. They also sort and organize those impulses, so that the messages are sent to the appropriate centers in the cerebral hemispheres. The thalamus probably has a role in discriminating between pleasant and unpleasant sensations and in the mechanism for arousal (alertness). It also registers crude touch and pressure sensations.

The Hypothalamus. This center is much smaller than the thalamus; it weighs less than 14 grams. It is connected to the rest of the CNS and to the pituitary gland. The pituitary gland is an endocrine gland that is known as the "master gland" of the endocrine system. The activity of this important gland is regulated by the hypothalamus, so the tiny hypothalamus could be called the "master of the master gland." The hypothalamus secretes substances called **hormone-releasing factors**, which signal the anterior lobe of the pituitary gland when it should release its hormones into the circulation. It also functions partly as an endocrine gland, secreting two hormones that are then stored in the posterior pituitary gland. These hormones are **oxytocin (OCK-see-TOH-sin)** and **antidiuretic (AN-tih-DYE-yoo-RET-ick) hormone (ADH)**. Oxytocin stimulates the smooth muscle in the walls of the uterus during childbirth. Its role in males is not understood. ADH is a hormone that regulates the balance of fluid in the body by regulating kidney function.

The hypothalamus has other important

roles as well. The most crucial of these is regulation and coordination of the autonomic nervous system. This is the system that controls the involuntary muscle activities of digestion, blood circulation, and other vital activities of the internal organs. The hypothalamus stimulates and inhibits the activities of the **viscera (VIS-er-ah)** or internal organs as needed. It also regulates appetite, telling the body when it is hungry and when its need for food is satisfied.

The hypothalamus, because it links the cerebral hemispheres with the autonomic nervous system, provides the link between emotions and the internal organs. For example, when the body is too hot, the hypothalamus directs the flow of blood to the skin surface to radiate heat out through the skin. But the same response that causes a reddening of the skin also occurs when a person is embarrassed or angry. Thus, the same physical response may be known as either a "flush" or a "blush" depending on the original cause—but both are regulated by the hypothalamus. The same principle applies to visceral emotional responses such as diarrhea or constipation in times of stress.

The Cerebrum or Cerebral Hemispheres

The cerebrum is the largest part of the brain. It is divided into two halves, which are called the cerebral hemispheres (or half-circles). Both halves are covered with a layer of gray matter called the **cerebral cortex (KOR-tecks)**. This layer is only about 2 to 4 mm thick, but it is arranged in folds or convolutions to fit as much of it into the enclosed space of the skull as possible. It contains 10 to 14 billion neurons and synapses, making it the most integrated and complex portion of the nervous system. In contrast, the brains of lower animals with less sophisticated intelligence than humans

TREATING FLUID RETENTION

A diuretic is a drug that increases urine production. This can be useful in treating fluid retention associated with congestive heart failure, a condition in which the heart's ability to pump blood is decreased. Increasing the urine output helps decrease fluid retention in the lungs, making it easier for the patient to breathe.

have smooth surfaces.

The folds in the cerebral cortex divide the brain into sections. The two halves are divided by a deep fold called the **longitudinal fissure (FISH-yoor)**. The cerebrum and cerebellum are divided at the **transverse fissure**. Then each hemisphere is further divided into lobes by shallower folds: the central sulcus **(SUL-kus)**, lateral sulcus, and parieto-occipital sulcus. The lobes themselves are named after the skull bones that are above them: the **frontal**, **parietal**, **temporal** and **occipital lobes**. One additional section of the cortex is the insula **(IN-syoo-lah)** which is inside the lateral fissure and can only be seen by spreading the fissure open or by dissecting the brain.

The two halves of the brain are not completely separate in spite of these fissures and sulci. The longitudinal fissure is bridged in the center by a band of white fibers called the **corpus callosum (KOR-pus kah-LOH-sum)**. Thus, the two hemispheres have a means of communication.

Below the cerebral cortex is a mass of bundles of white matter consisting of nerve fibers. Buried within this network of nerve tracts are masses of gray matter called **basal ganglia**. There are four of these centers in each cerebral hemisphere. These ganglia, which are also called the **cerebral nuclei**, are joined to each other, to the cerebral cortex, and to the spinal cord. This network is part of the system that links the higher brain to the motor neurons in the spinal cord.

All of these parts of the human brain work

together to create the complex mechanism that is *Homo sapiens* or humans. This includes the ability to move at will, to function internally without conscious effort, and also to exist as an intelligent, intellectual, communicating creature. The ability to speak and to react based on experience (i.e., the ability to learn) especially differentiates humankind from other animals. The cerebral cortex is responsible for the integration of sensation and response that makes these sophisticated processes possible. The white fibers in the cerebrum are also critical to these functions because they transmit messages back and forth throughout the central nervous system. Let us look briefly at how this system works.

Areas of the Cerebral Cortex

The cortex is divided into areas that contain specific functions of the brain (see Figure 10). In general, these specific areas cross the longitudinal fissure, so that part of each one is found in both the left and right sides of the brain. Almost all the neurons that transmit impulses from these areas to produce actions by the rest of the body cross each other, either in the medulla oblongata (part of the brain stem) or in the spinal cord. As a result, impulses that originate in the right hemisphere of the brain cause actions on the left side of the body, and the left hemisphere produces movement on the right side of the body. That does not mean there is no communication between the two hemispheres; remember that the corpus callosum connects the two.

The major areas of the cerebral cortex are the **primary motor area, premotor area, motor speech area, prefrontal area, general sensory area, auditory (AW-dih-TOH-ree) area, visual area,** and **olfactory and gustatory (GUS-tah-TOH-ree) area** (see Table 3 for the functions of each area). The remainder of the cortex consists of **association areas**. The association areas integrate input and responses.

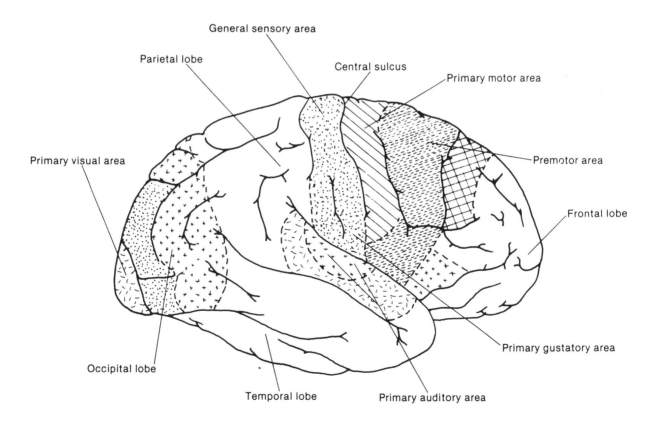

Figure 10: The cerebrum, illustrating sensory and motor areas.

Table 3: Functions of Areas of the Cerebral Cortex

Area	Functions it Controls
Primary motor	Voluntary, fine movements, as of hands and fingers, lips, tongue, vocal cords; precise muscle contractions
Premotor	Coordinates large autonomic skeletal muscle activity such as maintaining posture, chewing, swallowing, swinging the arms when walking, hand gestures with conversation
Motor speech	Forming words for both speaking and writing
Prefrontal	Complex intellectual activities such as planning, problem-solving, control of behavior
General sensory	Discrimination of sensations, as in recognition of shapes and textures and comparisons of intensity of sensations
Auditory	Hearing sounds
Visual	Receiving visual impulses
Olfactory	Receiving odors
Gustatory	Receiving flavor sensations

The two halves of the cerebrum are not identical, but all these major areas except the motor speech area are represented on both sides. In most people, one hemisphere or the other dominates. This is indicated partly by right- and left-handedness. Remember, the neurons cross each other, so a left-handed person has a dominant right hemisphere and a right-handed person has a dominant left hemisphere. In most people, the centers for speech and language are located on the left side. A few left-handed individuals, however, have those centers in the right hemisphere.

The right and left hemispheres have different overall functions (see Figure 11). The left side usually is responsible for analytic, logical, and language functions, whereas the right side governs musical and artistic skill and appreciation, simple words and mathematical calculations, intuition, imagination, space and pattern perceptions, and physical activity. This difference was first discovered when patients with apparently incurable epilepsy were treated by an operation in which the surgeon severed the connection between the hemispheres (the corpus callosum). Many of these patients continued to function normally in most respects, and their seizures were controlled. However, the lack of communication between the sides of the brain left some instructive gaps. For example, they were unable to describe actions of the left hand (which are controlled by the right hemisphere) because the speech center is on the other side of the brain. But they were able to demonstrate memory of the event by repeating the same motion when told to do so.

The Limbic Cortex. The **Limbic (LIMB-bick) Cortex** is the part of the cerebral cortex that has been called the "emotional brain" or the "visceral brain." It is located around the edges of the cortex at the corpus callosum and is connected with the hypothalamus and one of the basal ganglia. It is believed that this area of the brain contains memories of past experiences, especially those related to pain, pleasure, odors, and sexual activity. This information is combined with incoming sensations, and responses are relayed to the body through the hypothalamus to cause behavior such as excitement, rage, or sexual stimulation. Tranquilizers appear to act on the limbic cortex of the brain, reducing excitability and anxiety.

Sleep, Wakefulness, and Consciousness. Sleep and wakefulness are controlled by a system within the brain known as the **reticular (reh-TICK-yoo-lar) activating system** or **reticular formation**. This system consists of small islands of gray matter joined by bundles of fibers. It extends from the spinal cord to the cerebral cortex through the center of the brain stem and passes through both the hypothalamus and the thalamus. Stimulation of this system causes waking and/or heightened alert-

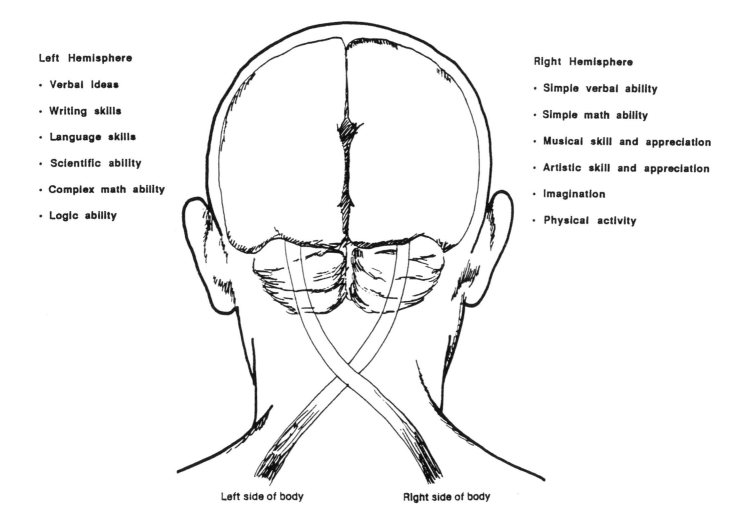

Left Hemisphere

- **Verbal Ideas**
- **Writing skills**
- **Language skills**
- **Scientific ability**
- **Complex math ability**
- **Logic ability**

Right Hemisphere

- **Simple verbal ability**
- **Simple math ability**
- **Musical skill and appreciation**
- **Artistic skill and appreciation**
- **Imagination**
- **Physical activity**

Left side of body   Right side of body

Figure 11: Functions of the right and left hemispheres of the cerebral cortex.

ness. Damage to this part of the brain causes unconsciousness or coma. In a coma, a person cannot be aroused.

Sleep is a state between alertness and unconsciousness in which the systems of the body slow down and the body and mind are at rest. There are several levels of sleep. **Rapid eye movement (REM) sleep** and **non-rapid eye movement (NREM) sleep** or **slow-wave sleep (SWS)** are the best known. REM sleep is almost always associated with dreaming and more active brain waves [as recorded by **electroencephalography (ee-LECK-troh-en-SEF-ah-LOG-rah-fee) (EEG)**]. NREM sleep includes four stages, which also can be identified through EEG recordings of brain waves. These levels (REM and NREM) alternate during normal sleep. Both kinds of sleep have been found to be essential for mental and physical health, although individuals may need differing amounts of sleep to function at their best.

Memory, Learning, and Acquired Reflexes. Animals function almost entirely on the basis of reflexes or instincts with which they are born. A mother cat with her first litter somehow knows how to raise her young; a duckling knows how to swim. Humans also have many inborn reflexes and instincts, but our behavior is controlled in large part by what we remember of what we have experienced or what we have been taught. For example, infants urinate whenever their bladder fills up. But as children grow up, they learn how to control the urinary sphincter. At first, this basic body func-

> ## IMPROVING THE MEMORY
>
> The ability to remember facts and events improves if the material to be remembered is used repeatedly over a long time. ""Cramming" for tests may help students get through an exam, but there will be little longterm retention of the material. Likewise, explaining medications and self-care issues to patients only once will often not be enough. Repeating the instructions each time the patient is seen in the office and giving printed reminders may help increase compliance with medical advice.

tion is an unconscious, involuntary activity. Then the child learns to control it, and the function comes under the regulation of the cerebral cortex. The same principle applies to learning to eat with a knife and fork, getting dressed, or tying shoes. These functions are difficult at first but eventually become almost automatic, even though they are under our conscious control.

The process by which the brain stores and retrieves such learned behavior and also other kinds of memories is not fully understood, although it is known to have both chemical and electrical components. There is some question of whether the human brain is in fact capable of fully understanding its own function—it is far more complex than the most sophisticated computer yet designed. We do know that memories can be either short-term or long-term. They are stored in association areas of the cerebral cortex as **engrams (EN-gramz)** or **memory traces**.

Short answer

1. Name the three parts of the brain stem.

    a. _____

    b. _____

    c. _____

2. Explain the function of the cerebellum.

    _____

    _____

3. Name the three parts of the diencephalon.

    a. _____

    b. _____

    c. _____

Matching

4.   Match the number of the area of the cerebral cortex next to the function it controls.

Cortex

1. olfactory

2. prefrontal

3. visual

4. general sensory

5. motor speech

6. auditory

7. premotor

8. primary motor

9. gustatory

Function

a. receives odors

b. discrimination of sensations, such as recognition of shapes and textures and comparisons of intensity of sensations

c. receives flavor sensations

d. hears sounds

e. voluntary fine movements, as of hands and fingers, lips, tongue, and vocal cords; precise muscle contractions

f. forms words for both speaking and writing

g. coordinates large autonomic skeletal muscle activity such as maintaining posture, chewing, swallowing, swinging the arms when walking, hand gestures with conversation

h. complex intellectual activities such as planning, problem solving, and control of behavior

i. receives visual impulses.

THE PERIPHERAL NERVOUS SYSTEM

The peripheral nervous system provides information to the CNS in the form of sensations and also carries out the directions of the CNS through the cranial nerves and the spinal nerves. This part of the nervous system can be divided into several areas for study: **sensory** or **afferent nerve pathways** which gather data in the form of sensations; **motor** or **efferent nerve pathways**, which stimulate action, movement or change; and the autonomic or **visceral system**, which controls involuntary activity in the internal organs.

Let us look first at the concept of **sensation**. Sensation can be defined as a state of awareness of external and internal conditions of the body. Sensation is necessary for survival. The environment, both external and internal, is constantly changing and the organism must change with it to maintain the steady state required to function. More specifically, sensations consist of combinations of input from sensory nerves. For example, a pinprick on the skin causes pain and a sensation of pressure. It also stimulates sensory nerves that help the brain identify the exact location of the source of pain. All these pieces of information are necessary for the removal of the problem.

A sensation has four components. It must be received by a receptor, converted into a nerve impulse, conducted to the brain, and translated from an impulse to a specific sensation by the appropriate area of the brain.

Receptors are found in the dendrites or cell bodies of sensory nerves. They can be classified in several ways. If they are grouped by location, there are three main classes:

- **Exteroceptors (ECKS-ter-oh-SEP-torz)** conduct impulses from outside the body (e.g., temperature changes, pain generated from the outside environment, vision, hearing, etc.). They are found in the skin, connective tissues, and parts of the gastrointestinal tract.

- **Visceroreceptors (VIS-er-oh-ree-SEP-torz)** pick up messages from within the body, such as the signal that food is being swallowed. They are found in organ tissues.

- **Proprioreceptors (PRO-pree-oh-SEP-torz)** are found in muscles, tendons, and joints. They detect muscle tone, movement of muscles and joints, and body position.

If receptors are grouped by the type of stimulus they detect, they can be classified as follows: **mechanoreceptors (MECK-ah-noh-ree-**

SEP-torz), thermoreceptors (THER-moh-ree-SEP-torz), nociceptors (NOH-see-SEP-torz) (pain receptors), electromagnetic receptors, and chemoreceptors.

Pain receptors are found in almost every body tissue except the brain itself. An adequate stimulus for a pain receptor is the extreme of any type of stimulus: cold, heat, pressure, tension, and so forth. Pain is the emergency signal of the sensory nervous system.

Unlike other sensations, pain is not lost by adaptation of the nerves. Adaptation means that the sensation is not registered by the brain even though the stimulus continues. For example, the body adapts to smells and sounds that persist over time, so that you no longer notice their presence. Pain can be inhibited by drugs, acupuncture, and surgical treatment in which the sensory nerve is severed. There are also some naturally occurring pain-relieving substances in the body—a type of chemotransmitter that inhibits pain impulses. For example, endorphins, which are CNS neurotransmitters that are chemically similar to morphine, raise the pain threshold, reducing pain and producing natural sedation.

Pain that occurs in an internal organ is sometimes referred to an area of the skin. That area may be near the site of the pain or away from it. One well-known example is angina or heart pain, which is caused by loss of circulation to the heart. It may be felt not only in the chest above the heart, but also along one or both arms.

Pain may sometimes be "felt" in a limb that has been amputated—that is, the limb is no longer there. This phenomenon is known as **phantom pain**.

Sensations occur at several different levels related to their destination in the CNS. Some reach only the spinal cord, and the response is a simple reflex. Others reach the lower part of the brain stem; these cause more complex sub-

conscious motor reactions. Impulses that terminate in the thalamus reach consciousness, but their origin in the body can only be located generally. Sensations that reach the cerebral cortex can be located with much more precision. Millions of minor and major adjustments are constantly made by the nervous system without conscious awareness of them. These occur at the spinal cord level, and in the brain stem. The sensations that stimulate these adjustments are carried by the **sensory nervous system**, and the unconscious responses are carried out by the **autonomic nervous system**. The input we are conscious of also comes from the sensory nervous system, but the conscious responses we make are made through the **somatic nervous system**. All three are part of the peripheral nervous system.

Particular types of sensations follow specific nerve pathways. For example, pain and temperature information from all parts of the body follow the **lateral spinothalamic (SPYE-noh-thah-LAMICK) pathway** up the spinal cord to the thalamus. Crude touch and pressure follow the **anterior spinothalamic pathway**, which travels to the same destination (the thalamus) but by a different nerve bundle in the spinal cord.

Responses also follow specific pathways. For example, voluntary muscle movements of the somatic system follow the **pyramidal (pih-RAM-ih-dal)** and **extrapyramidal (ECKS-trah-pih-RAM-ih-dal)** pathways from the motor cortex in the cerebrum to the spinal cord and from there to the appropriate effectors. These pathways cross over from one side of the brain to the other side of the body, either at the pyramids in the brain stem or in the spinal cord.

The Autonomic Nervous System

This division of the peripheral nervous system was once thought to be autonomous (not connected to the rest of the nervous system), which explains its name. In fact, the autonomic system is monitored and controlled by the central nervous system, just as the somatic system is. The major difference is that autonomic functions are not consciously willed—they occur automatically. The cerebral cortex, hypothalamus, and medulla oblongata are all involved in the control of the autonomic nervous system.

Visceral Effectors.   The effector neurons of this system are known as visceral effectors. They control cardiac muscle of the heart, smooth muscle, and glandular tissues. Smooth muscle is found in the blood vessels, bronchial tubes, stomach, gallbladder, intestines, bladder, spleen, some parts of the eye, and the hair follicles in the skin. Glands controlled by this system include the **lacrimal** (tear) **glands**, sweat glands, digestive glands (salivary, gastric, pancreas), and the adrenal medulla.

The autonomic system can either stimulate or inhibit these muscles and glands. It has two sets of neurons: the **sympathetic**, which stimulate, and the **parasympathetic (PAR-ah-SIM-pah-THET-ick)**, which inhibit.

Sympathetic Neurons.   The sympathetic neurons originate in two chains of ganglia, one on either side of the spinal cord. The nerve fibers that attach them to the cord are from the thoracic and lumbar regions, so the sympathetic system is also called the **thoracolumbar (THO-rah-koh-LUM-bar)** system. Nerve fibers that lead to these ganglia are known as **preganglionic (PREE-gang-glee-ON-ick) fibers** and those that leave the ganglia are called **postganglionic (POST-gang-glee-ON-ick) fibers**. Preganglionic fibers from the spinal cord terminate in the chain, and postganglionic fibers either go directly to effectors or join the spinal nerves and branch out from there.

These neurons are responsible for a set of automatic reactions to stress known as the **fight or flight syndrome** (see Figure 12). When under a stress such as fear, the body prepares for maximum exertion, whether it be to fight

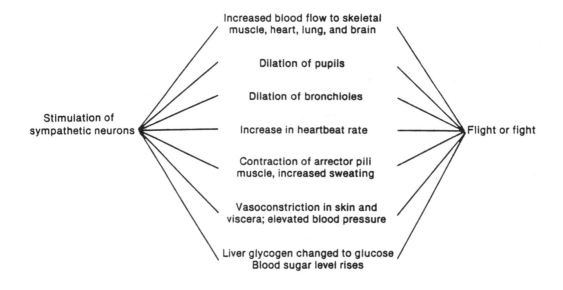

Figure 12: Flight or fight syndrome.

against the perceived threat or to flee from it. Sympathetic reactions include: increased heart rate; increased sweating; dilation of the pupils of the eyes; constriction of the blood vessels in the skin; elevated blood pressure; contraction of the muscles that control the hairs in the skin; dilation of the bronchioles in the lungs; increased blood flow to brain, heart, lungs, and skeletal muscles; and conversion of glycogen to glucose in the liver to increase the blood-sugar level.

Parasympathetic Neurons. The parasympathetic neurons originate in ganglia called **terminal ganglia**, which are located in the walls of the visceral organs. Preganglionic fibers for these centers come from the brain (cranial nerves) and the sacral region of the spinal cord. The parasympathetic division of the autonomic system is responsible for conservation and resto-

ration of energy and elimination of wastes. Unlike the sympathetic system, it does not cause a series of coordinated reactions. Instead, it often affects one organ at a time.

The effects of parasympathetic stimulation include the following: contraction of muscles in the bronchioles to slow breathing; contraction of the walls of the stomach, intestines, and bladder to increase their activity; inhibition of the salivary glands and heart rate; relaxation of the sphincters in the digestive tract and bladder; stimulation of secretions by the stomach and pancreas; and stimulation of a particular type of thin, watery saliva in the salivary glands.

To review the effects of the two divisions of the autonomic nervous system, look at Table 4 and Figure 13. Notice that many organs are affected by both divisions but with different and even opposite results.

Table 4: Examples of Effects of Sympathetic and Parasympathetic Stimulation

Effector	Sympathetic	Parasympathetic
Heart	Increases rate and strengthens beat	Reduces rate only
Bronchial tubes	Dilates	Constricts
Iris of eye	Dilates (enlarges pupil size)	Constricts (reduces pupil size)
Blood vessels	Constricts (usually)	No effect (in most cases)
Sweat glands	Causes secretions	No effect
Intestines	Reduces activity	Stimulates activity and secretions
Liver	Stimulates conversion of glycogen to glucose	No effect

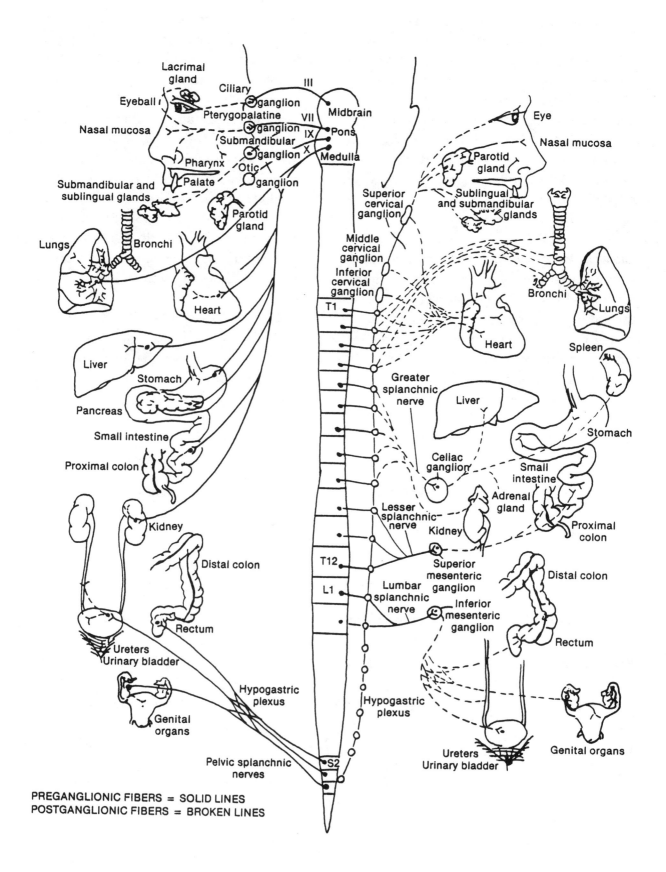

Figure 13: Autonomic nervous system; left side illustrating parasympathetic division, right side illustrating sympathetic division. Each division actually occurs on both sides.

Short answer

1. Name the four components of a sensation.

   a. _____

   b. _____

   c. _____

   d. _____

2. Name four reactions controlled by the sympathetic nervous system.

   a. _____

   b. _____

   c. _____

   d. _____

3. Name four reactions controlled by the parasympathetic nervous system.

   a. _____

   b. _____

   c. _____

   d. _____

True or False

4. Pain receptors are found in the brain. T/F

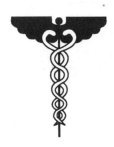

Knowledge Objectives

After completing this chapter, you should be able to:

- explain several tests used to diagnose neurological disorders
- name and describe several treatments used for neurological disorders, including (where appropriate) drugs and surgical methods
- list and describe the common symptoms of neurological diseases
- describe the symptoms of and treatment for transient ischemic attacks and strokes
- describe the types, symptoms, and treatment of brain hemorrhage
- describe the symptoms and treatment of brain and spinal cord injuries and tumors
- describe the symptoms of and treatment for epilepsy
- describe the symptoms of and treatment for infections of the nervous system, including meningitis, encephalitis, poliomyelitis, rabies, and shingles
- describe the symptoms of and treatment for functional disorders, including Bell's palsy, cervical spondylosis, carpal tunnel syndrome, Guillain-Barré syndrome, cerebral palsy, and hydrocephalus
- describe the symptoms of and treatment for degenerative diseases, including Parkinson's disease, multiple sclerosis, Friedreich's ataxia, and Alzheimer's disease

CHAPTER 2

Diseases of the Central Nervous System

INTRODUCTION

Some nervous system disorders are easy to identify as being caused by physical damage, inflammation, infection, and so forth. But neurological symptoms are sometimes caused either partially or completely by psychological disorders or by stress. A good example of this is the headache. Headaches may be caused by physical problems such as brain hemorrhage, concussion, eyestrain, or **meningitis (MEN-in-JYE-tis)**, to name just a few possibilities. Other headaches result from sinusitis or other problems not related to the nervous system. Still others are the result of nervous tension, depression, anxiety, and other problems that will not be evident on **computerized tomography** (CT) scan, **magnetic resonance imaging** (MRI) or examination of the cerebrospinal fluid. To diagnose the cause of a headache, the physician must be able to assess a patient's mental and emotional state as well as his or her physical condition. This requires painstaking observation of the patient and a detailed knowledge of nervous system function.

The tools of diagnosis for neurological problems include such varied equipment as a straight pin, a tuning fork, hot and cold water, an electroencephalograph, a reflex hammer, and an ability to pick up subtle verbal and physical clues to emotional distress, disorientation, or memory loss. Treatment ranges from the intricacies of brain surgery (neurosurgery) to providing encouragement and intensive nursing care to a helpless patient while waiting to see which nerves will begin to function again after an injury. Occasionally, a couple of aspirin and a good night's rest are all that is needed for a complete cure.

In this chapter, we will look in more detail at some of the tools used to diagnose and treat nervous system disorders, followed by brief descriptions of some neurological symptoms and some of the most common neurological disorders.

DIAGNOSIS OF NEUROLOGICAL PROBLEMS

The diagnosis of neurological disease begins with a patient history to determine the chief complaint and present and past medical illnesses. A review of the body systems and a general physical examination are performed. A neurological examination is then conducted that may consist of the evaluation of mental status (intellect, recent and remote memory, emotional state, verbal skills, appropriateness of emotional state, and the presence or absence of hallucinations and delusions), presence and strengths of muscle groups, sensory examination (touch, pain, temperature, proprioception, vibratory), special sensory examination (vision, hearing, smell, taste), and reflex examinations (pupillary, deep tendon, superficial skin, proprioceptive, and abnormal reflexes such as the Babinski reflex). Frequently, further special tests are indicated, including MRI, nerve conduction, electroencephalograms, CT scans, nerve or brain biopsy, cerebrospinal fluid examination, and blood analysis for identification of pernicious anemia, hyperglycemia, hypoglycemia, thiamine or electrolyte deficiencies, and poisons.

As a result of the history and examination, a preliminary neurological diagnosis is made. This diagnosis is usually confirmed by the response to therapy or the clinical course.

Reflex Tests

Several reflexes can be tested quickly and easily to obtain general information about motor neuron function.

The Patellar Reflex. Also known as the knee-jerk reflex, this is tested by striking the patient's knee just below the kneecap or patella. Normally, the lower leg will automatically extend. This indicates a complete two-neuron reflex arecat the second, third, and fourth lumbar nerves and proper function of the related muscles.

The Babinski Reflex. The **Babinski (bah-BIN-skee)** reflex is tested by using a blunt object to stroke the outside of the sole of the foot. Normally, this causes the toes to flex immediately. An abnormal response occurs if the big toe extends and the other toes fan out. This is known as the **Babinski sign** and it usually indicates impairment of the spinocortical nerve pathways. However, the Babinski sign is normal in infants.

The Achilles Reflex. Also known as the ankle

jerk, the **Achilles (ah-KIL-eez)** reflex is similar to the patellar reflex. On tapping the Achilles tendon in the ankle, the foot should flex. The centers for this reflex are in the first and second sacral nerves.

The Corneal Reflex. This is demonstrated when the eye closes as the examiner touches the cornea. This reflex involves responses from the fifth cranial nerve, the pons, and the seventh cranial nerve.

The Abdominal Reflex. This reflex is initiated by stroking the side of the patient's abdomen. The normal response is a drawing in of the abdominal wall, and it is initiated by the ninth to the twelfth thoracic spinal nerves.

Other Tests

Once it is established that the patient may have a neurological problem, other tests can be used to pinpoint the problem. Only a few of the more important tests are described here.

Lumbar Puncture. In this procedure, also called a spinal puncture, a needle is inserted through the dura into the subarachnoid space at the level of the third and fourth lumbar vertebra. Because the spinal cord ends at the level of the second lumbar vertebra, the risk of damaging the spinal cord is minimal. However, care must be exercised to avoid penetrating blood vessels or damaging spinal nerves. Because of these hazards, this procedure should only be attempted by well-trained medical personnel.

The lumbar puncture is performed to measure pressure in the central nervous system and to obtain fluid for examination and laboratory testing. The fluid can be tested for blood, other foreign cells, infection, and chemical imbalances. The same technique is used to inject medications, anesthetics, or contrast media for x-ray studies (myelography) into the spinal canal.

Electroencephalography (EEG). This technique

is used for measuring the electrical activity of the brain. Electrodes are attached to the patient's skull and to a recording device that makes a tracing of electrical impulses from many areas of the brain. Characteristic patterns occur in specific disorders. For example, various forms of epilepsy cause particular brain-wave patterns on an EEG.

The EEG is a painless procedure. The patient should be awake, alert, and calm and should have eaten recently (hypoglycemia or low blood glucose levels can affect brain activity). Additional readings may be taken after the patient is asked to breathe deeply 20 times a minute for 3 minutes. This increases the alkalinity of the blood and may reveal abnormalities that are not apparent in ordinary circumstances. A reading may be taken with a stroboscope flashing in the patient's eyes to examine a patient with light sensitivity. Finally, an EEG reading may be taken while the patient is asleep to see if abnormalities are evident under those conditions.

The EEG can be used to determine brain activity for patients in a coma. A patient who has a "flat" EEG (i.e., one that shows no activity) and who has no reflexes, breathing, or muscle activity for 6 hours or more is considered dead, even if circulation can be mechanically maintained. This is because the brain tissue is almost all dead and cannot be regenerated. A flat EEG may occur in extreme hypothermia (body temperature below 70° F) or with high dosages of depressant drugs (barbiturates, for example).

Other abnormal EEG waves are known as **delta waves**, **theta waves**, and **spikes** or **sharp waves**. In certain combinations, these waves indicate epilepsy, EEGs can also be used to test for brain tumors or abscesses, subdural hematomas, cerebrovascular disease (circulatory problems in the brain), brain injuries, and

EEG PREPARATION

Because drugs affect brain functioning and therefore EEG patterns, many types of drugs (such as stimulants, tranquilizers, and anticonvulsants), should be withheld from the patient for 24 to 48 hours before the EEG test. The physician prescribing these medications should be consulted to ensure that withholding these medications will have no adverse effects on the patient's health. Patients should also be advised to abstain from caffeinated drinks (cola, coffee, tea) during this time.

coma or other changes in consciousness. The EEG can also be used in a technique called the **evoked response**. A particular part of the nervous system is stimulated, such as visual auditory, or sensory areas, and EEG readings are taken. The response of the brain to the stimulus can then be analyzed by the physician.

X-rays of the Skull and Spine. X-rays or **radiologic examination** of the skull or spine are used to diagnose injuries, tumors, and spondylitis (inflammation of the vertebrae).

CT Scans. Computerized tomography or CT scan has largely replaced pneumoencephalography (injecting air into the ventricles of the brain to visualize the structure) and in many cases provides better information than ordinary x-rays. The CT scan gives a clear picture of the ventricles, the subarachnoid space, blood clots, nerves, tumors, cysts, and the major fissures and sulci of the brain. The CT scanner produces a series of x-ray "slices" through the body that are then assembled by a computer. The procedure involves low risk for most patients and provides information that is difficult to obtain by any other method.

Angiography. Angiography (An-jee-OG-rah-fee) provides information about the condition of the blood vessels in the brain. A substance called a **radiopaque contrast medium**, which is designed to show up on x-rays, is added to an artery through a catheter. The progress of the medium can be observed through a series of x-rays or films. Blockages and narrowing of the arteries can be detected as the substance moves through the circulation. Ruptured or leaking vessels can also be seen. The carotid arteries in the neck are often the source of emboli (circulating blood clots) that enter the brain, so these vessels are examined with angiography when such problems are suspected.

Two angiograms are commonly performed to examine the blood flow to the brain. The **carotid arteriogram (ar-TEE-ree-oh-GRAM)** outlines the carotid arteries in the anterior neck and the anterior and middle cerebral arteries of the brain. The **vertebral arteriogram** demonstrates the vertebral arteries in the posterior neck, plus the posterior cerebral arteries of the brain.

Myelography. This procedure is used to demonstrate structures in and around the spinal cord. A needle is inserted into the spinal canal between the third and fourth lumbar vertebrae. Recall that the spinal cord ends at the level of the second lumbar vertebra and that lumbar punctures are performed at this level to avoid damaging the spinal cord. The physician injects a radiopaque contrast medium into the subarachnoid space. After taking a series of radiographs with the patient in various positions, the contrast medium is removed to avoid irritation of the meninges. **Myelography (MYE-eh-LOG-rah-fee)** can assess the size and position of tumors, ruptured intervertebral discs, and trauma to the spinal cord and spinal canal. A CT scan is in many instances able to provide the same information as the myelogram but with less discomfort to the patient.

Radiosotope Scan. In some cases, the techniques listed above fail to detect a tumor or blood vessel blockage. The radioactive isotope technique may succeed in locating the problem in such situations. Instead of an opaque substance, a radioactive substance is injected into the bloodstream. This substance is detected and measured as it localizes in the CNS. This is a more sensitive test than angiography.

MRI Scan. Using this procedure, it is possible

to look at soft tissue rather than bone or blood vessels. Thus, growths in white or gray matter are easier to detect than with other tests. Also, injections of either radioactive or radiopaque media are not necessary, which reduces the risks for the patient.

STOP AND REVIEW

Short answers

1. Describe the test and normal response for the following reflexes:

   a. patellar reflex _____

   _____

   b. Babinski reflex _____

   _____

   c. Achilles reflex _____

   _____

   d. corneal reflex _____

   _____

   e. abdominal reflex _____

   _____

2. Describe the purpose of the following procedures:

   a. lumbar puncture _____

   _____

   b. electroencephalography (EEG) _____

   _____

   c. x-rays of the skull and spine _____

   _____

   d. CT scan _____

   _____

e. angiography _____

_____

f. myelography _____

_____

g. radioisotope scan _____

_____

h. MRI scan _____

_____

TREATMENT OF NEUROLOGICAL DISEASES

The treatment for diseases of the nervous system can be divided into five major categories: prevention, rehabilitation, drugs, surgery, and braces and traction.

Prevention

Cerebrovascular (SER-eh-broh-VAS-kyoo-lar) accident or **stroke** (along with heart attacks is one of the most common causes of death in Western countries. Prevention of stroke is similar to the prevention of heart disease because the two problems have similar causes. High blood pressure and its companion problem, arteriosclerosis, are described in detail in the book in this series on the cardiovascular system. These diseases lead to stroke as well as heart attack, as both are caused by impaired circulation of blood to the brain and heart. Prevention may involve changes in diet (reducing salt, fats, and cholesterol); changes in life-style, especially quitting smoking and regular exercising; and treating high blood pressure with drugs. **Anticoagulant (AN-tih-koh-AG-yoo-lant)** drugs may be prescribed to prevent abnormal clots from forming.

Another type of neurological disorder that calls for preventive measures is injury to the brain or spinal cord. Such injuries cause many deaths and also leave many people severely handicapped. Prevention of such injuries involves ordinary common sense more than medical prescriptions. For example, wearing seat belts can prevent many head injuries. Accidents resulting from climbing shaky ladders, riding motorcycles without wearing helmets, and other careless acts can lead to major trauma or require extensive rehabilitation and can sometimes cause death. Patient education regarding routine safety precautions is one way the medical profession can help prevent injuries.

Drugs

A number of drugs that are used to treat other kinds of medical problems are also used in neurology.

- Pain medications or **analgesics (AN-al-JEE-zick)** are often needed. Once the source of pain has been identified, the patient needs pain relief to regain strength and allow for healing. Such drugs must be used with caution in brain injuries, however, because of the danger of depressing (decreasing) nervous system activity when it is already depressed by tissue damage.

- **Antibiotics (AN-tih-bye-OT-icks)** are prescribed to treat bacterial infections of the nervous system.

- Anticoagulants may be prescribed as a preventive measure for patients who are susceptible to strokes due to abnormal clot formation. One example of an anticoagulant is heparin, which is used to prevent clotting in intravenous lines in patients. Another anticoagulant is warfarin, which is given to patients to prevent the formation of thrombi (blood clots).
- **Vasoconstrictors (VAS-oh-kon-STRICK-torz)** may be helpful for migraine-like headaches caused by dilation of the blood vessels that supply the head or brain.
- **Vasodilators (VAS-oh-dye-LAT-orz)** such as nitroglycerin help relieve pain from angina pectoris or pain in the chest felt by patients with heart problems.
- **Antihistamines (AN-tih-HIS-tah-meens)** are sometimes prescribed for the same reason as steroids—to reduce inflammation in allergic reactions. One frequently prescribed antihistamine is diphenhydramine, which is used to treat reactions to be stings, poison ivy, and the contrast media used in radiology.
- **Antiemetics (AN-tih-ee-MET-icks)** or drugs that suppress nausea and vomiting may be prescribed when vomiting is a symptom of diseases such as meningitis. These drugs block nerve impulses from the inner ear to the vomiting center in the medulla oblongata. Dimenhydrinate (Dramamine) is an example of a drug used for this purpose.

Other drugs such as the following, may be prescribed specifically for their effects on the central nervous system.

- **Anticonvulsants (AN-tih-kon-VUL-sants)**, as their name implies, are prescribed to prevent convulsions or seizures. There are several different formulations that can stabilize the activity of the brain and combat the electrical disturbances that cause epileptic seizures Phenytoin, for example, is one anticonvulsant that is commonly used in the treatment of epilepsy. Some of these drugs have a sedative effect—that is, they may also cause drowsiness. They are some-

times prescribed in combination if a single drug does not effectively control seizures.
- **Antiparkinsonian (AN-tih-PAR-kin-SOH-nee-an)** drugs are used to treat Parkinson's disease. They initiate a complex chemical action that ultimately supplies missing chemotransmitters, which in turn correct the abnormal transmission of nerve impulses. Drugs used to treat Parkinson's disease include levodopa (L-dopa) and a combination of L-dopa with carbidopa.
- **Central nervous system depressants** are drugs that slow down the activity of the nervous system. Barbiturates constitute a major group of these drugs. They usually have a sedative or sleep-inducing effect such as that produced by thiopentalsodium, a drug sometimes introduced intravenously as an anesthetic. They also may be habit forming—that is, they can cause dependency in some patients, either physical (the patient builds up a tolerance for the drug and experiences withdrawal symptoms when it is not taken) or psychological (the patient feels a need for the drug, but no physical changes have occurred to make the drug physiologically necessary). These drugs may be given to halt a seizure (as in status epilepticus) or to help a patient sleep. They may be prescribed for psychological disorders as well.
- **Central nervous system** stimulants are drugs that accelerate nervous system activity. They may be prescribed to treat narcolepsy and aid in weight loss. They may also be helpful in treating hyperactive children.

Neurosurgery

Surgery is sometimes effective in correcting neurological problems. In the peripheral nervous system, where nerve fibers are capable of regeneration, the nerves themselves can sometimes be repaired. New techniques such as **microsurgery** (using a microscope to see tiny structures as they are being repaired) are employed to repair nerves and reattach severed fingers, toes, and even limbs.

In a few instances, surgeons are called upon to sever nerves rather than to repair them. For example, in some cases of duodenal ulcer disease, a portion of the vagus nerve is severed to reduce the production of stomach acid. Another example is surgery for relief from **tic douloureux (TICK doo-loo-ROO)**, a painful nervous disorder involving the seventh cranial nerve. If medical treatment fails, a neurosurgeon may be called upon to sever the nerve, resulting in paralysis of one side of the face.

More often, neurosurgery is needed to remove abnormal growths, drain abscesses or excess fluids, remove foreign objects (such as bullets or skull fragments), remove tissue that is pressing on a nerve, or repair ruptured blood vessels. All of these operations, especially when they involve the brain or spinal cord are extremely delicate procedures. Any error can result in permanent impairment of function or even personality. Stored memories can be wiped out with just a deviation of 1 micrometer in the surgeon's aim.

Neurosurgery is an extremely specialized field. For this reason, it requires several years of training under the supervision of highly trained experts in addition to the four-year residency required for most medical specialties.

Traction and Braces

Sometimes, a problem in the nervous system is caused by a pinched nerve or some other kind of physical pressure on a nerve. Such problems may be treated with a back or neck brace or by putting the patient in traction. Traction involves immobilizing a patient and using weights and braces to hold a limb or the spine in one position until healing occurs.

SYMPTOMS OF NEUROLOGICAL DISEASES

Some of the most common neurological symptoms are headache, numbness and tingling, and pain. Others include **photophobia (FOH-to-FOH-bee-ah)**, or extreme sensitivity to light; blurred or double vision; fainting; **coma**; paralysis; seizures; mental confusion; personality changes; mood disorders; and **aphasia (ah-FAY-zee-ah)**, **ataxia (ah-TACK-see-ah)**, and **apraxia (ah-PRACK-see-ah)**.

Headache

This symptom varies from minor complaint to disabling pain. It may be felt as a throbbing, stabbing, or dull ache. In attempting to identify the cause of a headache, the physician will elicit as detailed a description of the sensation as possible, including the time of day it occurs, how long it lasts, whether it seems to be focused on one place in the skull, any events that regularly precede or follow the headache (such as an encounter with the boss or a menstrual period), and so forth. Different causes of headache produce different characteristic forms of the symptom. For some patients, the analysis of headache pain is difficult because they consider headache to be a single symptom and assume all headaches are alike. Careful questioning and observation are helpful in obtaining detailed information in such cases.

Headaches may be caused by pressure on the brain, eyestrain, or pressure on the arteries that lead to the brain. Cutting into brain tissue is not painful because there are no pain receptors in that tissue. However, there are pain receptors on the surface of the skull and around the blood vessels and other structures of the brain. Also, when brain tissue is injured or infected, it swells like any other injured tissue (the inflammatory response). This puts pressure on the brain because it is in the enclosed cavity of the skull. Such swelling causes severe headaches. The same thing happens when a growth occurs on or in the brain—there is no room for expansion to accommodate additional tissue.

Numbness and Tingling

These symptoms often are an early indication of damage to the peripheral nervous system or to centers in the brain or spinal cord that govern the area where sensation is felt. They may be felt down one entire side of the body, in one limb, in the hands or feet, or in the face.

Pain

Pain can have many causes, some of which are merely carried by the nervous system and some of which occur because of disease or injury to the nerves. Examples of nervous system disorders that cause pain include pinched nerves; neuritis (inflammation of nerve tissue); **sciatica (sye-AT-ih-KAH)** (pinched or inflamed sciatic nerve that innervates the legs); and **shingles (herpes zoster)**, a disease caused by the chickenpox virus that results in inflammation of the spinal ganglia. The usual causes are damage to or pressure on the nerves or inflammation due to infection.

Photophobia

Patients sometimes describe a sensitivity to light that almost amounts to fear. This symptom occurs with infection of the brain such as meningitis. It may also be a symptom of brain hemorrhage.

Blurred or Double Vision

Several of the cranial nerves are involved with the process of focusing and otherwise adjusting the eyes to see clearly. Many different brain disorders, including stroke, transient ischemic attacks, tumors, and infection, can cause vision disorders in one or both eyes.

Syncope (SIN-koh-pee) or Fainting

Fainting or brief unconsciousness is caused by a momentary loss of adequate blood supply to the brain.

Coma

Coma is unconsciousness or complete lack of responsiveness that lasts more thant 2 or 3 minutes. The brain is functioning, but the patient cannot be roused to a waking state. Like faint-

---

FORMS OF AMNESIA

Although memory loss is the most familiar type of amnesia, this condition may take different forms depending which part of the brain is affected. For example, in visual amnesia a person cannot remember how to read. Auditory amnesia affects the person ability to understand the spoken word. Tactile amnesia prevents a person from recognizing a familiar object by touch.

---

ing, it is usually caused by a loss of circulation to the brain, often due to physical or chemical injury to the brain or a ruptured or blocked blood vessel. Unrelieved coma may result in brain damage or death.

Paralysis

This term means the inability to move some part of the body voluntarily. It may be temporary or permanent. When one side of the brain is damaged by a stroke, tumor, or injury, the opposite side of the body may become paralyzed.

Seizures

Other terms for this symptom are **fit** and **convulsion**. Seizures are caused by electrical abnormalities in the brain. There are many forms of seizures, ranging from the dramatic grand mal seizure in which the patient becomes unconscious and rigid and falls to the floor with repeated muscle spasms to incidents of momentary "absence," or petite mal seizures that may go completely unnoticed.

Mental Confusion

Disorders of the brain such as tumors and injuries can cause confusion. The patient may suddenly become forgetful of either recent events or the past. This is due to disturbances in the memory areas of the brain. Loss of memory of past events is called **amnesia (am-NEE-zee-ah)**. The patient my either be aware of the problem and very anxious about it or completely unaware of memory lapses. Another form of mental confusion is **disorientation**, in which the patient does not know where he or she is or cannot identify the year or the time of day.

Personality Changes and Mood Disorders

When the areas of the brain that control mood, emotions, or personality are damaged or bruised, the patient may become anxious, depressed, or elated, experience sudden mood changes known as **mood swings**, or exhibit a different personality than usual. Often the patient is unaware of such changes, and the altered behavior is reported by family or friends.

Aphasia

This term means inability to speak. It is caused by damage to the speech center in the cerebral cortex (usually in the left hemisphere). A person with aphasia may be able to understand oral and written communication but be unable to formulate words either to speak or to write. It can be very frustrating for the patient.

Ataxia

A person with ataxia cannot control voluntary muscle movements. This symptom may be caused by damage to the cerebellum or the motor area of the cerebral cortex.

Apraxia

This term means inability to carry out learned, voluntary actions such as dressing or eating, even though the patient wants to do them. It is the result of damage to memory centers in the cerebral hemispheres.

The next section of this chapter examines some of the specific diseases that can cause these symptoms.

STOP AND REVIEW

Short Answers

1. Name seven symptoms of neurological disease.

   a. _____

   b. _____

   c. _____

   d. _____

   e. _____

   f. _____

   g. _____

2. Name the five methods of treatment of neurological diseases.

a. _____

b. _____

c. _____

d. _____

e. _____

NEUROLOGICAL DISEASES AND DISORDERS

Stroke

Stroke is the common term for cerebrovascular accident (CVA). In a stroke, the circulation of blood to some part of the brain is interrupted. An artery may be blocked by an **embolus (EM-boh-lus)**, which is a blood clot or other circulating piece of material (air, fat, tumor cells). A vessel may be gradually blocked by **atherosclerosis (ATH-er-OH-sklee-ROH-sis)**, the development of deposits of cholesterol and other substances in the arteries. The interruption may be due to a burst blood vessel caused by an **aneurysm (AN-yoo-rizm)**, a weakness in the blood vessel wall. This is called a **cerebral hemorrhage**. The blood from the damaged vessel seeps into brain tissue, causing additional damage. Whatever the cause, the result is tissue death in the part of the brain that is no longer receiving a blood supply. The severity of the illness depends on how much and what part of the brain is damaged.

Symptoms. The symptoms of stroke may include numbness or heaviness of a limb, inability to move a particular limb or side of the body, inability to speak, headache, blurred or double vision, confusion, loss of memory, and sometimes loss of consciousness. A person who has had a stroke and cannot speak may be perfectly able to understand what is going on but be unable to formulate words (aphasia).

Diagnosis and Treatment. Stroke is diagnosed by the symptoms and by neurological examination, CT scan, and EEG. Treatment depends on the severity of the damage. The first priority in severe cases is to maintain or restore breathing and circulation. Surgery to repair damaged arteries or remove a blockage may be useful in some cases. Anticoagulants may be used in the case of emboli and thrombosis. Subsequent treatment is aimed at rehabilitation—helping the patient relearn lost skills and adapt to any permanent disability. This process may take a long time and require a great deal of patience, encouragement, and emotional support from health professionals and the patient's family and friends. The doctor may also recommend changes in diet and lifestyle to guard against future strokes.

Transient Ischemic Attacks

Some people have minor, temporary symptoms similar to those of strokes, such as momentary blackouts, temporary blurred vision or confusion, sudden but temporary blindness in one eye, and so forth. These may be warning signs that the circulation to the brain is in danger. Such warnings are called transient **ischemic (is-KEM-ick) attacks (TIAs)**. They occur when a cerebral blood vessel becomes blocked but is quickly reopened or bypassed by the circulatory system.

Diagnosis. A patient who reports such symptoms will be tested for circulatory system problems, including high blood pressure and heart disease. Test may include an electrocardiogram (ECG), carotid and cerebral angiography, carotid Doppler studies, and x-rays of both the heart and skull. The aim is to locate the sites of blockage or embolism formation.

Treatment. Treatment may include removal of **atheroma (ATH-er-OH-mah)** (deposits in the blood vessels) if the site of the problem allows for it and/or anticoagulant drugs to reduce the risk of clot formation. Aspirin may be all that is necessary, but in some cases stronger medications are required. The doctor will want to monitor the patient's progress and may also prescribe blood pressure medication, changes in diet, and/or changes in exercise and other habits. About 30% of patients experiencing a TIA will suffer a stroke within 5 years, so it is important to guard against this danger. For example, smoking contributes to the risk of stroke, and quitting smoking may be an important aspect of treatment.

Brain Hemorrhage

Bleeding in the brain can occur as the result of a fall or other injury or from a burst aneurysm. Cerebral hemorrhage is a form of stroke. The vessel ruptures inside the cerebrum and damages the brain tissue. A brain hemorrhage can also cause bleeding into the subarachnoid space, the subdural space, or outside the dura mater.

Subarachnoid Hemorrhage. This bleeding usually is caused by a burst aneurysm. The blood mixes with cerebrospinal fluid already in the subarachnoid space and may slowly seep into the brain tissue. Symptoms are sudden severe headache, a stiff neck, photophobia, and sometimes dizziness, confusion, nausea and vomiting, or loss of consciousness (coma). Death may follow. If the patient survives, there may be brain damage; there is also a risk of a second similar hemorrhage. Treatment may involve painkillers for the headache, surgery to repair aneurysms, blood pressure treatment, and rest. Arteriography (x-ray studies of the arteries using radiopaque contrast media) may be performed to locate possible sites of future problems. Patients may have partial paralysis, weakness, and other effects after an initial recovery.

Subdural Hemorrhage and Hematoma. The ruptured blood vessels in this type of brain hemorrhage are on the underside of the dura mater. The blood may gradually collect between the dura mater and the arachnoid layer and form a clot or hematoma **(HEM-ah-TOH-mah)**. This problem usually occurs after a head injury resulting in a broken or torn vein. Symptoms may not develop for several days or even weeks. They may include drowsiness, confusion, weakness or numbness on one side of the body, headache, or nausea. The symptoms may come and go, but they gradually worsen. The patient may not remember the fall that caused the injury—it may have seemed quite minor at the time. Treatment involves surgery to stop the bleeding and remove the blood. A portion of the skull may have to be removed and replaced to do this. Recovery is usually complete.

Extradural Hemorrhage. In this circumstance, the ruptured blood vessel is on the outside of the dura mater, and blood flows into the space between the meninges and the skull. Like subdural hemorrhage, this problem is usually caused by a head injury resulting in a broken or torn artery. The symptoms begin within 24 hours and include sudden severe headache, nausea, vomiting, and drowsiness that gradually deepens into coma. An extradural hemorrhage, also known as an epidural hemorrhage, is an emergency situation that can result in brain damage or death. Treatment is basically the same as for subdural hemorrhage.

Brain Injury

Most injuries to the brain that cause lasting damage occur in traffic accidents (especially those involving motorcycles), industrial accidents, explosions, or gunshot wounds. Whether the skull is fractured or not, a severe blow to the head can cause bruising, jolting, or other damage to the brain. The results of a brain injury depend on the force of the blow and which part of the brain is involved. A minor injury will cause headache that may last for several days. A more severe injury will cause unconsciousness lasting for a few seconds to several weeks. When the brain is bruised it tends to swell, and this causes pressure on the brain because the skull cannot expand with the brain tissue. The swelling along with possible breakage of the skull bones, may cause permanent damage. The brain is capable of healing, however. Although damaged cells cannot be regenerated, bruised cells may recover and other nerve cells can take over lost functions. However, this process may take a long time.

A person who has been in a coma from such an injury and who regains consciousness may be confused and disoriented. Loss of memory (amnesia) may occur. Headaches, weakness, paralysis, and problems related to specific cranial nerves or areas of the brain (such as vision problems and speech problems) may be present. Such problems may gradually improve or they may persist. It is difficult or impossible to predict the outcome of such injuries or how long it will take for the patient to recover. Later, seizures, depression, personality changes, and other symptoms may develop.

Important terms related to brain injury are **concussion** and **contusion**. A concussion **(kon-KUSH-un)** is a loss of consciousness with possible temporary impairment of brain function. A contusion **(kon-TYOO-zhun)** of the brain is bruising of brain tissue, which causes loss of consciousness and often is related to skull fracture. A contusion is more serious than a concussion.

Diagnosis and Treatment.. To assess brain injury, physicians use skull x-rays, CT scans, and arteriography. Steroid drugs may be given to reduce swelling. Although codeine may be prescribed, other pain medications such as morphine or CNS depressants are generally not prescribed because they may further depress brain function. Surgery to remove bone fragments or to repair other structures may be necessary. Further treatment consists of rest and a gradual return to as much normal function as possible with the help of physical therapists, occupational therapists, and other health professionals.

Spinal Cord Injuries

When the spinal cord is injured, the functions that are controlled by the nerves below that point are affected (see Figure 14). However, sometimes an injury will affect only one side of the body. Remember that the spinal cord contains the nerve pathways from the body to the brain. If that connection is severed, the spinal nerves can neither deliver nor receive messages and they become useless. The nerve cells in the spinal cord, like those in the brain, cannot regenerate; but, unlike the brain, the spinal cord does not have millions of extra cells that can take over the function of damaged cells. As a result, spinal cord injuries often cause permanent loss of function, including numbness, weakness, and paralysis. The symptoms of a spinal cord injury are evident immediately. In most cases, absence of sensation rather than pain predominates.

If the nerves that control breathing are damaged, a spinal cord injury will be fatal, unless someone at the scene keeps the patient breathing with artificial respiration. These nerves are in the neck. Injuries lower on the cord may not be fatal but often produce permanent disability. The nerves that control the bladder and rectum also stem from the spinal cord and are often affected.

Treatment. It is very important to avoid moving a person who may have a spinal cord injury. Special equipment designed to keep the spine immobilized must be used. If the person is moved incorrectly, damage to the cord may be worsened. Once the patient reaches a hospital, damage can be assessed by neurologic examination and by x-rays of the spine, CT scan, MRI, and myelography. Surgery will be attempted if broken or displaced bone or other tissue around the nerves can be repaired. The patient will then probably have to spend several months in the hospital. With time and rest, some nerve tissue that is not actually severed

or dead may recover. Otherwise, treatment focuses on preventing bedsores and infections (especially bladder and kidney infections), assisting with bowel and urinary function, and rehabilitation. Patients may be paralyzed from the neck down, including the arms (**quadriplegia (KWOD-rih-PLEE-jee-ah)**), from the waist down (**paraplegia (PAR-ah-PLEE-jee-ah)**), or on one side (**hemiplegia (HEM-eh-PLEE-jee-ah)**). These patients can learn to manage amazingly well if they are generally healthy and determined and if they receive help and encouragement from medical professionals, family, and friends.

Brain or Spinal Cord Tumors
Tumors of the central nervous system are uncommon. The most common form is second-

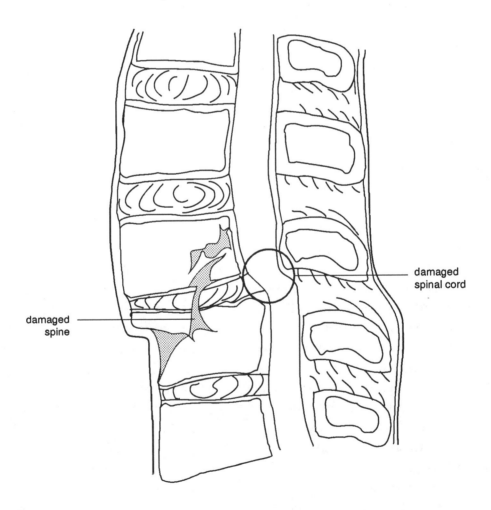

damaged spine

damaged spinal cord

Figure 14: Fracture of lower cervical spine with damaged spinal cord.

ary cancers that have spread from cancer sites elsewhere in the body, most often from the lungs or breast. A tumor in the brain or spinal cord may be benign or malignant (cancerous), but both are very serious because they cause pressure on nerve tissue. In the brain, there is no extra room within the skull for a tumor to grow, so it will grow into the soft tissue of the brain itself. In the spinal cord, the vertebrae also form a nonexpandable compartment, and any abnormal growth will sooner or later press on the bone and/or the nerves.

Symptoms. General symptoms of brain tumor are frequent severe headaches, nausea and vomiting (and sometimes sudden vomiting without nausea), seizures, and blurred or double vision. Other symptoms depend on the location of the tumor and may include weakness on one side, unsteadiness, loss of the sense of smell, memory loss, and sometimes personality change. Spinal cord tumors cause back pain. Depending on the location of the tumor, numbness, coldness, weakness in specific limbs, or problems with urination or defecation may occur.

Diagnosis and Treatment. Tumors of the central nervous system are diagnosed by x-rays, CT scans, MRI scans, angiography, and/or radioisotopic scans in the brain and by x-rays, CT scans, MRI scans, and myelography in the spinal cord. Treatment consists of removing the tumor surgically and/or by radiation treatment or chemotherapy. In some cases, pressure can be temporarily relieved by removing part of the tumor, or in the spinal cord, by chipping away part of the vertebra. Steroid drugs may be prescribed to reduce swelling, and surgery may be followed with radiation treatment.

Benign tumors that have not penetrated deeply into nerve tissue can often be removed completely with no after effects. Malignant brain tumors are more difficult to treat suc-

cessfully. A patient with a malignant brain tumor seldoms lives longer than 1 year, even with surgery, radiation, or chemotherapy.

Epilepsy

Epilepsy is a malfunction of the electrical activity of the brain that causes periodic seizures. By definition, epileptic seizures occur more than once. They may occur in response to a particular stimulus such as a bright light or stress, but more commonly they occur with no particular pattern. There are many different forms of this disease and many different types of seizures. Some common types of seizures are listed in Table 5.

Epilepsy can be the result of brain damage cause by disease or injury or it may be a symptom of brain tumor. It can also be an inherited disorder. Some seizures first appear at the time of puberty and may be associated with increased hormone levels circulating in the blood. In many cases, however, the cause is unknown and no damage is visible in the brain to explain why the seizures occur. Nevertheless the seizures are the result of abnormal electrical impulses in the brain, and these can be recorded on an EEG.

Diagnosis and Treatment. Epilepsy is diagnosed by a description and history of seizures and by examining EEG tracings. Each form of the disease has its characteristic pattern of brain waves. Treatment is with anticonvulsant drugs which the patient should take regularly to prevent seizures. Such treatment is often very effective. The drugs may have side effects, especially if they are taken in large doses, so patients may be tempted to stop taking them and will then have seizures again. Some patients need to take anticonvulsants indefinitely, but in some cases, especially when the seizures started in childhood and have no apparent cause, the drugs can be gradually withdrawn when the patient has been seizure-free for several years and the EEG no longer shows seizure activity.

Handling Seizures. Most epileptic seizures are not harmful in themselves, although a person having a grand mal seizure may be injured by fall or crashing into furniture. If you are present while someone is having such a seizure, the best thing to do is to move potentially harmful ojects out of the way, while avoiding interference with the person's movements. Trying to prevent the person from swallowing his or her tongue is *not* recommended, and in general nothing can be done to prevent the twitching and jerking. However, there is a disorder known as **status epilepticus (STAY-tus ep-ih-LEP-tih-kus)** that is dangerous and should be considered a medical emergency. In this condition, the patient has several seizures in rapid sequence, with no time for recovery in between. The treatment of status epilepticus begins with making sure that the patient is breathing and then injecting drugs to depress the nervous system and/or sedate the patient until the seizures stop.

Table 5: Types of Seizures

Type	Description
Grand mal	Can occur at any age. The patient falls down unconscious, goes rigid, twitches or jerks rhythmically, and may urinate, then slowly regains consciousness. Seizures are usually followed by deep sleep or confusion. May be preceeded by an aura or warning sign consisting of vision problems, or numbness.
Petit mal	Occurs in childhood. The child suddenly goes blank for up to 30 seconds and does not know what is happening. After the seizure has passed, he or she probably will not know it occurred.
Focal seizure	Uncontrollable twitching that begins in one part of the body such as the thumb, followed by twitching of the surrounding structures, then one side of the body, then the whole body. The patient is conscious during the seizure.
Temporal lobe seizure	After a brief warning or aura, the patient suddenly acts out of character for a few minutes with anger or laughter for no particular reason or some bizzare action. An unconscious chewing motion may occur during the seizure.
Febrile convulsion	Occurs during feverish illnesses in childhood. Similar to a grand mal seizure. An isolated convulsion is not a sign of epilepsy and should not cause any lasting damage to the nervous system.

Short answers

1. Name five symptoms of a stroke.

   a. _____

   b. _____

   c. _____

   d. _____

   e. _____

2. A transient ischemic attack is a sign that the patient is at risk for what neurological disease? _____

3. Name three types of brain hemorrhages.

   a. _____

   b. _____

   c. _____

4. Name three kinds of permanent loss of function caused by spinal cord injuries.

   a. _____

   b. _____

   c. _____

5. Name three symptoms of a brain tumor.

   a. _____

   b. _____

   c. _____

6. Define epilepsy and describe a method of diagnosis. _____

   _____

7. Name the five types of seizures.

   a. _____

   b. _____

   c. _____

   d. _____

   e. _____

INFECTIONS OF THE NERVOUS SYSTEM

Meningitis

This disorder is a viral or bacterial infection of the meninges, the covering of the brain. It often occurs as a complication of a viral illness such as the flu (influenza) or a complication of sinusitis or a severe ear infection. The symptoms are fever, headache, photophobia, nausea and vomiting, a stiff neck, and sometimes a rash. In severe cases meningitis can lead to drowsiness, unconsciousness and eventually death or blindness, but is not always a dangerous condition. It is diagnosed by analysis of the cerebrospinal fluid. Treatment is with antibiotics, **antipyretics (AN-tih-pye-RET-ick)** (antifever drugs), bed rest, and fluids if the infection is bacterial. Viral forms usually are less dangerous and are treated essentially the same way, except that antibiotics are usually not prescribed.

Encephalitis

Encephalitis (EN-sef-ah-LYE-tis) is inflammation of brain tissue, usually due to a viral infection. It may be a complication of mumps or measles. The disorder causes fever, headache, loss of energy, and sometimes irritability, restlessness, drowsiness. Loss of function such as muscle weakness, vision problems, temporary aphasia, and occasionally coma may also oc-

POLIO IMMUNIZATIONS

Even though polio is uncommon today, it is vital to maintain immunization for children. The American Academy of Pediatrics recommends that children receive a trivalent oral polio vaccine (TOPV) at age 2 months, 4 months, 18 months, and just prior to beginning school (between 4 to 5 years of age).

cur. Encephalitis is diagnosed by CT scan, EEG, and analysis of the cerebrospinal fluid. It may take several weeks or longer of bed rest, extra fluids, and possibly intravenous feeding before the patient recovers. In a few cases, the brain may be permanently damaged by the disease and death may occur.

Poliomyelitis

This disease, commonly known as **polio (POH-lee-oh)**, is a viral infection of the anterior horns of the spinal cord. It is uncommon today because a vaccine against it is readily available. It can cause permanent paralysis or muscular weakness in severe cases. The location of the damage in the spinal cord determines which muscles are affected.

Epidural Abscess

An abscess **(AB-ses)** is a pocket of infection marked by the collection of pus. Such an infection occurs rarely in the brain from an untreated bacterial infection. It is treated with antibiotics and perhaps surgical drainage. The abscess may be on or in the brain around the spinal cord.

Rabies

Rabies is a viral infection of the central nervous system spread by the bite of infected animals. It is rare today because most domestic animals are vaccinated against it. However, wild animals occasionally transmit it to unvaccinated pets or to humans.

Preventive treatment of suspected rabies is based on immunization with a series of vaccine and immune serum injections. When bites are in areas close to the head or in areas with many nerve endings such as hands, the virus may reach the brain very quickly. In such cases, treatment should start immediately even though the suspected animal is still being observed.

Agents used to confer passive immunity are human rabies immune globulin (HRIG) and antirabies serum, equine (ARS). Active immunity to rabies can be conferred by administration of human diploid cell vaccine (HDCV). This medication is injected five times over a 28-day period.

There is no cure for rabies once the symptoms appear. Treatment is palliative and includes sedation of the patient and provision of a quiet environment to reduce anxiety and relieve pain, administration of muscle relaxants, and supportive measures to maintain urinary and respiratory function.

Shingles

Shingles is a viral infection of the peripheral nerves that is caused by the same virus that causes chickenpox. It occurs only in patients who have had chickenpox. Apparently, the virus remains dormant in the body after the patient recovers from chickenpox and may erupt as shingles years later for no known reason. Sometimes the attack can be related to stress

SIGNS OF RABIES IN ANIMALS

Everyone (but particularly children) should learn to recognize the signs of an animal infected with rabies. Infected animals pass through several stages:

1. Wild animals often become very friendly encouraging children to approach and pet them;
2. Next animals enter a "furious" stage, biting everything within reach, both moving and stationary;
3. The throat muscles become paralyzed, making it difficult swallow. Animals appear to avoid water, giving rise to the term "hydrophobia";
4. Respiratory and other muscles become paralyzed, resulting in the death of the animal.

or injury, but in other cases no cause can be found. The symptoms are severe pain in the infected nerve and a blistery, itchy rash resembling chickenpox along the path of the peripheral nerves. It usually affects a nerve or nerves on one side of the trunk, but it can occur anywhere. Shingles can cause temporary facial paralysis or vision problems if nerves that supply the face and cornea of the eye are involved. It cannot be cured, but it eventually resolves on its own. Treatment is aimed at relieving the pain and itching. It may take several weeks or months to recover.

Reye's Syndrome

Reye's (RYEZ) syndrome almost always arises within 1 to 3 days of an acute viral infection, such as an upper respiratory infection, influenza, or chickenpox. It may be linked to aspirin use, and may cause encephalopathy and cerebral edema (swelling). However, if detected early, Reye's syndrome is not usually fatal.

Symptoms vary with the five stages of the disease. In early stages, the patient experiences vomiting, lethargy, changing mental status (including agitation, confusion, irritability, and delirium), rising blood pressure, increased respiratory and pulse rates, and hyperactive reflexes. In later stages, the disease may lead to coma, followed by seizures, decreased tendon reflexes, and respiratory failure.

Tests used to detect Reye's syndrome include liver function studies, liver biopsy, CSF analysis, coagulation studies, and blood tests. Early treatment includes intravenous fluids, a diuretic, and vitamin K. Later treatment may include intubation, mechanical ventilation, and drugs or other measures to reduce intracranial pressure.

Lyme Disease

This disease is caused by a **spirochete (SPYE-roh-keet**; spiral bacterium). It occurs when an infected tick injects saliva into the bloodstream or deposits fecal matter on the skin.

Lyme disease usually progresses in three stages. Initially, the patient may experience a persistent sore throat and dry cough. Then a hot, itchy lesion forms at the site of the tick bite. More lesions may erupt within a few days, as well as a rash, conjunctivitis, or wheals. Within 3 or 4 weeks, small red blotches replace the lesions and persist for several more weeks. Symptoms include malaise, fatigue, headache, fever, chills, achiness, and swollen lymph glands. The second stage begins several weeks later. Neurologic abnormalities develop, such as fluctuating meningoencephalitis and peripheral and cranial neuropathy, and usually resolve in several days or months. Facial palsy may also develop. The third stage, marked by profound and possibly chronic arthritis, begins weeks or years later.

Diagnosis hinges on detection of the initial lesion and related symptoms. Blood tests and liver enzyme tests may support the clinical diagnosis. The recommended treatment for adults includes 10 to 20 days of antibiotics, such as oral tetracycline, penicillin, or erythromycin.

Epstein-Barr Virus (EBV) Infection

Epstein-Barr virus (EBV) infection may be transmitted by exposure to infected saliva or blood products. The infection is known to cause infectious **mononucleosis (MON-oh-NYOO-klee-OH-sis)**, which produces headache, malaise, and fatigue for 3 to 5 days, followed by fever, sore throat, and swollen cervical glands. In rare cases, it may lead to complications, such as meningitis, encephalitis, and Guillain-Barré syndrome. EBV infection may also be linked to some forms of cancer, lymphoproliferative syndrome (Duncan's syndrome), and congenital infections.

EBV may be detected by serum antibody testing. Additional tests may reveal alterations in liver enzyme levels and increased white blood cell levels. Treatment is aimed at symptom relief and includes bed rest, antipyretics, and analgesics.

Chronic Fatigue Syndrome

The cause of **chronic fatigue syndrome (CFS)** is still unproven, but this neuropsychological disorder may be related to EBV infection. It usually follows an accute infection, such as respiratory or gastrointestinal illness, flu-like disease, or bronchitis, and may be triggered by stress. The CFS patient will recover from the initial illness, but experience recurrent or constant symptoms of the disease for more than 6 months afterward. Patients primarily feel fatigue, weakness, and depression. Other symptoms include chills or low-grade fever, sore throat, tender lymph nodes, headache, joint pain (without swelling), and inability to concentrate and perform routine tasks.

There is no definitive test to detect CFS. However, tests may be used to detect elevated liver enzymes and immune system abnormalities that are commonly associated with the disorder, such as high levels of antibodies, circulating immune complexes, decreased gamma globulin production, and decreased natural killer cell activity.

There is no specific treatment for CFS. Different patients may respond to different treatments. For some patients, antidepressant drugs may be helpful. Others may find releif from alternative therapies, such as meditation, acupuncture, acupressure, and yoga. Most people recover completely from CFS, but the length of time required varies.

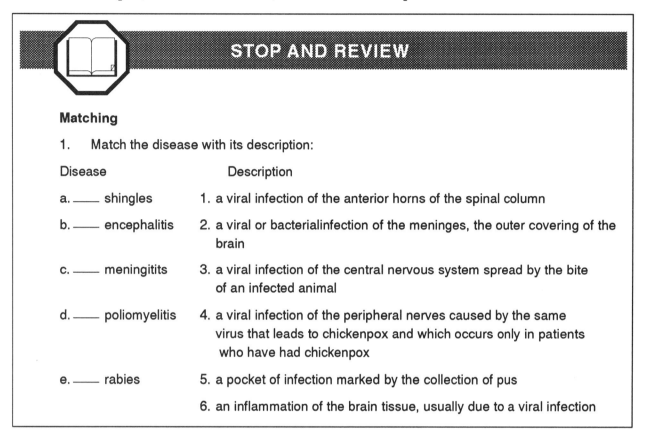

STOP AND REVIEW

Matching

1.   Match the disease with its description:

Disease	Description
a. ____ shingles	1. a viral infection of the anterior horns of the spinal column
b. ____ encephalitis	2. a viral or bacterialinfection of the meninges, the outer covering of the brain
c. ____ meningitits	3. a viral infection of the central nervous system spread by the bite of an infected animal
d. ____ poliomyelitis	4. a viral infection of the peripheral nerves caused by the same virus that leads to chickenpox and which occurs only in patients who have had chickenpox
e. ____ rabies	5. a pocket of infection marked by the collection of pus
	6. an inflammation of the brain tissue, usually due to a viral infection

STRUCTURAL AND FUNCTIONAL DISORDERS

Bell's Palsy

In this disorder, the facial nerve on one side swells for no known reason and becomes pinched where it passes through the skull. This causes muscle weakness on that side of the face, resulting in a distorted expression, a downward turn to the mouth, and sometimes an inability to close the eye. This condition is almost always temporary, but while it exists the eye must be protected against irritation because the lid can no longer close. The lid both protects the eye from injury and distributes tears on the surface of the eye to keep it moist. **Bell's palsy (BELZ PAWL-zee)** may last for 2 weeks to 2 months. In some cases, steroid drugs may speed recovery. Other treatment consists

of moistening the affected eye regularly and keeping it covered with a patch.

Cervical Spondylosis

The term **spondylosis (SPON-dih-LOH-sis)** means immobility of the vertebral joint. In this disorder, the vertebrae in the cervical region (the neck) develop bony growths. The discs between the vertebra may harden as well, and the whole structure of the neck may become stiff and misaligned. This creates abnormal pressure on the spinal cord and the spinal nerves that supply the arms and hands. The symptoms are a stiff neck, numbness and tingling, and/or pain in the hands and arms. In severe cases, the pressure affects nerves below the neck, causing muscle weakness in the legs and possibly bladder and bowel problems. It can put pressure on the blood vessels that supply the brain, which may cause dizziness, headache, or double vision. This condition can also occur in the lumbar spine.

Diagnosis and Treatment. The problem is diagnosed by x-rays, MRI, CT scan, and myelography. It is treated with a neck brace—a hard plastic collar in the daytime and a soft one at night. The doctor may prescribe a mild analgesic and muscle relaxant drugs. If the symptoms continue after about 3 months of wearing a supportive collar, traction and/or surgery to remove the excess bone may be recommended.

Carpal Tunnel Syndrome

The **carpal (KAR-pal) tunnel** is a rigid passageway between the carpal bones of the wrist and the ventral ligaments. Nerves from the brain to the hand pass through this tunnel. If the tissue in it becomes swollen from accumulated fluid, pressure on the nerves causes **carpal tunnel syndrome**. The symptoms are tingling and numbness in the hand and shooting pains that travel from the wrist up the arm, usually at night. Carpal tunnel syndrome is most commonly found in post-menopausal women and may be attributed to repetitive motions such as those involved in typing. Treatment may include a splint worn on the affected wrist at night, diuretic drugs to reduce fluid in the body, and steroid drugs to reduce inflammation. If these measures are not effective, surgery may be necessary to free the nerve and create more space in the carpal tunnel.

Peripheral Neuropathy

This term refers to damage to the peripheral nerves. It can be caused by chronic disorders such as diabetes or alcoholism, by a deficiency of vitamin B_{12}, by taking certain drugs such as aspirin in large quantities for many years, or from overexposure to a toxic substance such as arsenic, mercury, or lead.

Symptoms. The problem appears gradually in most cases, beginning with tingling in the hands and feet that spreads up the limbs to the trunk. Numbness may then develop, following the same pattern. Sensitive skin and nerve pain may also occur, followed by muscle weakness. Numb areas of the body may become injured and ulcers may form. Also, dexterity is reduced; this can lead to accidents. Muscle weakness can eventually become paralysis.

Treatment. There is no cure for this disease; however, the process may be slowed or even halted if the cause can be removed. A diabetic person, for example, may be able to stop the progress of the disease, at least temporarily, by keeping more strictly to a prescribed diet and monitoring blood-glucose levels more carefully. Patients with **peripheral neuropathy (nyoo-ROP-ah-thee)** should be advised to watch for sores or bruises, especially on the hands and feet, and have them treated by a physician. Such apparently minor injuries heal poorly, may not be felt by the patient because of the damaged nerves, and can lead to gangrene (dead tissue).

Guillain-Barré Syndrome

This is a form of peripheral neuropathy that comes on suddenly rather than gradually. It usually occurs within 1 to 3 weeks of a viral infection or after immunization for a viral illness. Some scientists believe **Guillain-Barré (gee-YAN bar-RAY)** syndrome may be an autoimmune disease. Tingling, numbness, weakness, and sometimes paralysis occur in rapid sequence within a few hours. However, in most cases the symptoms eventually disappear. In cases where paralysis occurs, the patient may have to be hospitalized and sometimes needs a respirator to aid with breathing until the symptoms improve. Physical therapy may be needed to restore full function.

Migraine

Migraine (MYE-grayn) is a disease in which

the patient has periodic debilitating headaches. The headaches may be accompanied by nausea, vomiting, or blurred vision. In many cases, each headache is triggered by a factor such as ingestion of a particular food (e.g., cheese, chocolate, alcohol, caffeine, or a substance used as a food preservative), a stress situation, or the menstrual cycle, but in other cases no such factor is found. Physiologically, the pain and other symptoms are probably due to constriction of the arteries to the brain followed by dilation of those arteries, which disturbs normal blood flow to the brain. The headache is usually preceded by a warning signal called an **aura (AW-rah)**. This may be irritability, nausea, or a disturbance of vision such as blurred or double vision. The characteristics of the headache itself vary from patient to patient, but the pain is severe enough to keep the person from doing anything for a period of time ranging from several hours to a day or longer.

Treatment. For some patients, resting in a darkened room for several hours as soon as the warning aura begins can reduce the severity and length of an attack. Sometimes, drugs such as vasoconstrictors or antihistamines can have the same effect if they are taken when the aura begins. In severe cases, a doctor may prescribe a drug such as propranolol that the patient takes regularly to prevent migraines from occurring. If migraines are associated with menstruation and fluid retention, a diuretic may be prescribed. Because aspirin is a vasodilator, it is not effective against migraine. Another preventive measure is biofeedback, a technique in which the patient learns to voluntarily control blood vessel diameter by receiving feedback from a machine each time the desired result is obtained.

Cerebral Palsy

Cerebral palsy is caused by brain damage that occurs during fetal development, during birth, or in early childhood. One of more limbs may be immobile or weak, and muscle movements may be poorly controlled or jerky. These problems may be accompanied by mental retardation, but this is not always the case. Other possible problems are hearing loss, visual problems, speech problems, and convulsions. Cerebral palsy usually is not detected until a child is 6 months of age or older, when normal development calls for more coordinated muscle movements. Children with cerebral palsy may develop slowly in many areas, especially if they cannot move around to explore their environment or if visual or hearing problems limit stimulation.

Treatment. Damage to the brain cannot be repaired, but it should be carefully assessed so that all the child's abilities will be developed as much as possible. For example, deafness can be misinterpreted as retardation in an intelligent child, and thus a whole range of potential abilities may be neglected. Treatment for cerebral palsy includes physical therapy, speech therapy, special education, and other measures to maximize the child's ability to function. Physical therapy can sometimes enable wheelchair patients to learn to walk. Occasionally, surgery can be performed to reduce muscle stiffness. Vision and hearing problems can also be corrected or improved in some cases. Progress may be slow, even in patients with normal intelligence, because of the damage to the brain, but much can be accomplished with determination, patience, and constant support and encouragement for the child and his or her parents from family, friends, and health professionals.

Hydrocephalus

Hydrocephalus (hye-droh-SEF-ah-lus), or water on the brain, is an enlargement of the head caused by the presence of excessive cerebrospinal fluid (CSF). It is mainly a congenital (present at birth) condition and may be caused by inadequate absorption of CSF or by blockage of the ventricular system. Hydrocephalus occurs in four of every 1,000 infants between birth and 3 months of age. It is treated by surgically placing a shunt (tube) to drain the excess CSF from the ventricles. Patients must be closely observed after surgery for the signs of infection and obstruction of the shunt.

STOP AND REVIEW

Short answers

1. Name the cause and describe the symptoms of Bell's palsy.

   _____

   _____

2. Name three symptoms of cervical spondylosis.

   a. _____

   b. _____

   c. _____

3. Describe the symptoms of peripheral neuropathy.

   _____

   _____

4. Define and describe Guillain-Barré syndrome.

   _____

   _____

5. Describe the symptoms and progression of migraine headaches.

   _____

   _____

DEGENERATIVE DISEASES

Parkinson's Disease

This disease is also called **paralysis agitans (pah-RAL-ih-sis AJ-ee-tanz)**. It occurs because of deterioration of the basal ganglia and diminished supplies of the neurotransmitter chemical dopamine. This imbalance causes shaking and rigidity in the voluntary skeletal muscles. The patient has characteristic involuntary movements called **tremors**, such as rhythmic shaking of the head and hands or a pill-rolling movement in which the thumb and fingertips are rubbed together. The tremor goes away when the patient voluntarily moves the limb. The condition gradually worsens, and the patient may become unsteady and unable to write or speak clearly. The risk of accidental falls increases as the disease worsens. Parkinson's disease is not life-threatening because it does not affect the autonomic nervous system. However, it can eventually lead to deterioration of memory and intellect, and patients may become depressed by their inability to control ordinary movements. Treatment with drugs that increase the amount of dopamine in the brain can significantly improve the symptoms of Parkinson's disease but cannot stop the progress of the disease or reverse the damage already done to the nervous system.

Multiple Sclerosis (MS)

In this disease, the myelin sheaths that cover the axons of many nerves (the white matter of the nervous system) become inflamed. The first (and in some cases the only) attack of the disease may cause a number of different symptoms, depending on which nerves are affected. It may cause numbness, tingling, or weakness in one or more limbs or in a single spot, ataxia, blurred vision, slurred speech, or urinary incontinence. These symptoms may be very minor and last only a few weeks. The disease usually appears between the ages of 20 and 40. A period without symptoms, called **remission**, follows the first attack. Later attacks may become gradually more frequent and/or more severe over a span of 20 to 30 years.

Diagnosis and Treatment. Multiple sclerosis (sklee-ROH-sis) is difficult to diagnose because the symptoms are so variable. EEGs and an analysis of the CSF may provide useful indicators. CT and MRI scans may also be ordered to rule out other causes of the symptoms. The disease cannot be cured, but the symptoms can sometimes be relieved with steroid drugs, muscle relaxants, or physical therapy during attacks. Incontinence is treated with a catheter in severe cases, but infections of the urinary and respiratory systems frequently occur. In about a third of the cases, multiple sclerosis leads to severe disability. In other cases it causes only minor disability or does not return for many years.

Amyotrophic Lateral Sclerosis (Lou Gehrig's Disease)

Amyotrophic lateral sclerosis (ah-MYE-oh-TROF-ick LAT-er-al sklee-ROH-sis) or ALS is a motor neuron disease that causes muscle atrophy. It affects men four times more frequently than women. The disorder may be inherited or may result from an autoimmune disorder or a metabolic disturbance.

Symptoms of ALS include fasciculations (**fah-SICK-yoo-lay-shunz**; small muscle contractions that are visible through the skin), atrophy, and weakness of the hand and forearm muscles. Other symptoms are impaired speech; difficulty chewing, swallowing, and breathing; choking; and excessive drooling.

ALS can be diagnosed through electromyography and muscle biopsy to identify nerve—rather than muscle—disease. The diagnosis may be supported by CSF analysis that shows increased protein levels.

Because ALS has no effective treatment, therapy aims to control symptoms and provide emotional, physiological, and physical support. The disease is usually fatal within 3 to 10 years of its onset.

Huntington's Chorea

Chorea (koh-REE-ah) means uncontrollable, jerky body movements. In this rare inherited disease, nerves degenerate in various parts of the body, usually starting between the ages of 30 and 45. Chorea and mental deterioration result. There is no cure and no effective treatment for the symptoms. Genetic counseling is the key to eventual eradication of this disease.

Friedreich's Ataxia

This is also an inherited disease, but it affects children beginning between the ages of 5 and 15. It also causes degeneration of nerve fibers, resulting in ataxia followed by problems with speech, arm movements, and even standing. It also causes heart disease. There is no known treatment for the disorder.

Chronic Organic Brain Syndrome

Chronic organic brain syndrome describes a broad range of senile dementia (decreased intellectual ability) in older adults. When this condition occurs before age 65, it is called **presenile dementia** or **Alzheimer's disease**. The symptoms are gradual loss of intellectual ability, memory, and other thought processes due to the death of nerve cells in the frontal and temporal lobes of the cerebrum. This disease progresses more rapidly in younger patients and eventually causes death.

Treatment. There are many possible causes of mental deterioration other than Alzheimer's disease, and many of them are treatable. It is important for any patient with such symptoms, regardless of age, to be tested for other possible causes of the problem. Some of these possibilities are nutritional disorders such as vitamin B_{12} deficiency, brain tumors, brain hemorrhage, and severe depression.

Table 6: The Central Nervous System and Drug Abuse

All drugs can be abused. Some categories of prescription drugs that can be overused with serious consequences for the patient are listed below, with the usual reason(s) for prescribing them and some of the dangers associated with them.

Category of Drug	Prescribed for	Dangers/Abuse
Amphetamines (am-FET-ah-minz) (stimulants)	Weight loss, hyperactivity	Used to increase wakefulness; can cause physical dependence; overdose can cause death
Barbiturates (bar-BIT-yoo-rayts) (sedative-hypnotics)	Sleeplessness, anxiety, digestive tract problems	Can cause physical dependence; overdose can cause death, especially when combined with alcohol
Methaqualone* **(meh-THAH-qwah-lohn)** (hypnotics)	Sleeplessness	Physical dependence; convulsions; death
Antianxiety drugs	Anxiety	Physical dependence; coma; death from overdose
Minor tranquilizers	Anxiety; to relax muscles	Psychological dependence; physical dependence in large doses
Analgesics (narcotic forms)	Pain	Physical dependence; convulsions; death from overdose

*Methaqualone is especially dangerous because tolerance to the drug increases the amount needed to achieve the desired effect (i.e., sleep), and the toxic level is relatively low. Thus, a patient may eventually "need" a toxic dose, and death may follow.

Some other drugs that affect the central nervous system are listed below:

Illegal
Heroin (narcotic analgesic)
Cocaine (stimulant)
LSD (stimulant)
Marijuana (stimulant)

Legal
Caffeine (stimulant)
Nicotine (stimulant)
Alcohol (depressant)

If the patient does in fact have Alzheimer's disease, no treatment is possible. Eventually, close supervision and nursing care will become necessary. Most Alzheimer's patients need intensive care provided by a nursing home because they lose the ability to take care of their own basic needs. Caring for such patients requires a combination of patience, gentleness, and firmness. Persons with Alzheimer's disease may not remember to eat or may forget that they have just eaten. Simple tasks such as dressing and going to the bathroom become very difficult, yet the patient may be able to walk and talk and may make unreasonable demands. The patient may also be angry at the situation and feel very helpless. This combination can result in an extremely difficult patient.

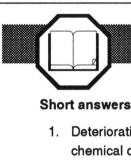

STOP AND REVIEW

Short answers

1. Deterioration of the basal ganglia and diminished supplies of the neurotransmitter chemical dopamine are the main causes of what disorder? _____

2. Name four symptoms of multiple sclerosis.

   a. _____

   b. _____

   c. _____

   d. _____

Matching

3. Match the disease with its description:

Disease

a. ____ Huntington's chorea

b. ____ Amyotrophic lateral sclerosis

c. ____ Friedreich's ataxia

d. ____ Alzheimer's disease

Description

1. A condition in which motor neurons die for no known reason

2. An inherited disease affecting children between the ages of 5 and 15, it causes degeneration of the nerve fibers resulting in ataxia and then problems with speech, arm movements, and even standing; it often also affects the heart

3. A disease that usually occurs in the elderly but which can begin in middle age; it causes gradual loss of intellectual ability, memory, and other thought processes and is the result of the death of nerve cells in the brain

4. A rare, inherited disease in which nerves degenerate in various parts of the body, starting in early middle age and causing uncontrollable, jerky body movements and later mental deterioration

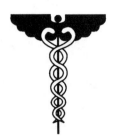

Knowledge Objectives

After completing this chapter, you should be able to:

- name the five special senses
- list and describe the structure of the gustatory and olfactory sensors
- describe the structure of the eye
- describe the structure of the ear
- describe the equipment used to diagnose and treat ear and eye disorders, including the ophthalmoscope, Snellen chart, audiometer, hearing aid, impedance testing, and electrocochleography
- describe the symptoms and treatment of eye disorders and diseases, including problems of refraction, infection, and inflammation and structural disorders
- describe the symptoms and treatment of ear and balance disorders, including hearing loss, blockages, and infections

The Special Senses

The special senses include taste, smell, vision, hearing, and the sense of position or balance. Their function is to give the brain information about the world outside the body, and involve specialized structures of the nervous system. They are discussed separately because they have complex sensory organs unlike any others in the nervous system.

TASTE AND SMELL

These senses are technically known as the **gustatory** (taste) and **olfactory** (smell) **senses**. The two are closely related because much of what we think of as taste is actually a function of smell.

Gustatory Sensors

The receptors for taste are located mostly on the tongue and on the soft palate (see Figure 15). They are known as the taste buds. Most of the taste buds are located in raised areas on the tongue called the **papillae (pah-PIL-ee)**. They are constructed from two kinds of cells— **supporting cells** and **gustatory cells**. The gustatory cells have microscopic hairs, and there are gustatory pores in the papillae above the hairs.

For a substance to be tasted, it must first be dissolved in saliva. It then flows through the gustatory pores and stimulates the hairs on the surface of the gustatory cells. Sensa-tions from the taste buds travel to the brain from the gustatory cells via cranial nerves VII, IX, and X (the facial, glossopharyngeal, and vagus nerves). They are interpreted in the medulla oblongata, thalamus, and cerebral cortex.

The gustatory cells can detect only four "tastes": sweet, salt, sour, bitter. Each taste bud specializes in detecting one of these flavors, and tastes buds are grouped in specific regions on the tongue. Each region has a few buds that pick up other tastes besides the one it specializes in. Beginning at the tip of the tongue and moving to the back, the regions are located in this order: sweet, salt, sour, and bitter.

Olfactory Sensors

The receptors for the olfactory sense are found in the mucous lining of the upper part of the nasal passages or the **nasal epithelium (EP-ih-THEE-lee-um)**. In the epithelium are olfactory cells, which contain dendrites of sensory neurons called **olfactory hairs**. The neurons convey impulses to the olfactory nerves, and from there they travel to the olfactory bulb in the brain. The olfactory tracts of the first cranial nerve convey these impulses to the cerebral cortex.

Supporting cells and glands surround the olfactory cells in the nasal lining. The glands secrete fluid that dissolves gases from odorous substances. Odors can only stimulate the sen-

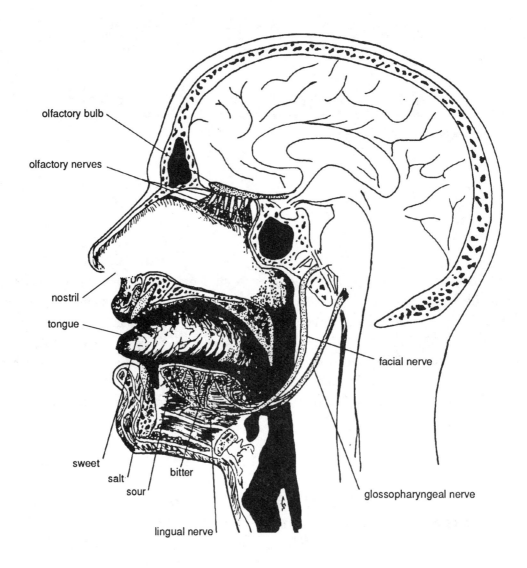

Figure 15: Organs of taste and smell.

sory nerve endings in the olfactory cells when they are in the form of dissolved gases. However, most people need only a very small amount of substance in the air to detect an odor. The olfactory cells adapt quickly to smells that persist but also pick up new scents quickly. Irritating odors such as the smell of ammonia stimulate the trigeminal nerve (fifth cranial nerve) as well as the olfactory nerve and cause pain. Thus, irritating odors should not be used to test the function of the olfactory nerve except to detect feigned or exaggerated symptoms.

VISION

The eye is a complex organ that collects light rays, focuses them into an image, and converts that image to sensory information for the brain to interpret.

Structure

Each eye is set in a cavity in the skull known as the **orbit** (see Figure 16). The eye itself takes up only a fifth of the space in the orbit. Behind it are muscles, nerves, blood vessels, and a cushion of adipose or fatty tissue. The eyelids or **palpebrae (PAL-peh-bree)** are protective curtains of skin and muscle that move up and down in front of the eyeball and are edged with hairs known as eyelashes. There are sebaceous glands in the follicles of the eyelashes and in the lids. The lids are lined with mucous a membrane called the **conjunctiva (KON-junk-TYE-vah)**. The **lacrimal (LACK-rih-mal) glands** are located on the outside upper edge of each eye. These glands secrete tears, a salty fluid designed to keep the surface of the eye moist and clean. At the corner of each eye closest to the nose are the **lacrimal duct** and **lacrimal sac**. These structures collect tears after they cross the surface of the eye and drain the fluid into the nasal passages. This is why a person's nose will run when the eyes tear.

Eye Muscles. Six different muscles move the eye in its orbit and anchor it in place. They include the four rectus muscles—**superior, inferior, medial**, and **lateral**—and the **superior** and **inferior oblique** muscles. With all these muscles plus the function of vision, it is easy to see why the eyes are related to so many cranial nerves (see Table 1, p.21).

Eyeball. The eyeball itself consists of three layers of tissue surrounding a transparent center (see Figure 17). The outer layer is called the **sclera** or the white of the eye. In the front of the eye, this layer changes in character and becomes the transparent **cornea**. The cornea allows light to enter the eye.

The second layer includes the **iris**, which lies below the cornea and in front of the lens. It has an opening in its center known as the **pupil**. The iris itself consists of a sphincter muscle and dilator muscle that work to open and close the pupil, regulating the amount of

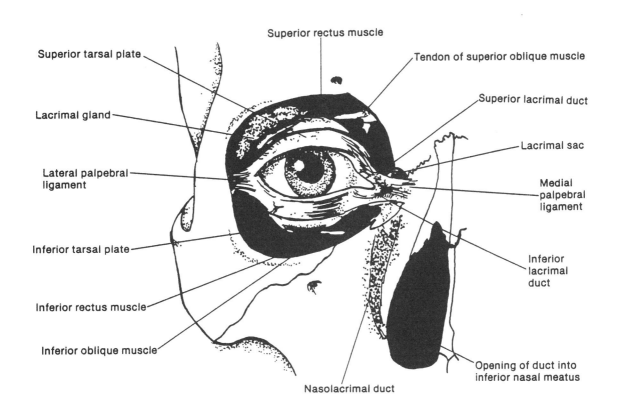

Superior rectus muscle
Superior tarsal plate
Tendon of superior oblique muscle
Lacrimal gland
Superior lacrimal duct
Lateral palpebral ligament
Lacrimal sac
Medial palpebral ligament
Inferior tarsal plate
Inferior rectus muscle
Inferior lacrimal duct
Inferior oblique muscle
Opening of duct into inferior nasal meatus
Nasolacrimal duct

Figure 16: The eye, anterior view.

light that enters the eye. The other parts of this layer are the **choroid layer**, the **ciliary (SIL-ee-ER-ee) body**, and the **ciliary muscle**. The ciliary muscle controls the curvature of the lense to adjust vision.

The third layer is the **retina (RET-ih-nah)**, which lines the interior of the eyeball. This layer includes the photoreceptors known as the **rods** and **cones**, specialized cells that are sensitive to light. The optic nerve enters the back of the eye and spreads out in transparent branches over the retina in order to pick up the impulses from these photoreceptors.

The interior of the eye is transparent, and contains several structures and chambers. Below the cornea and the iris is the **lens**, which is made of transparent protein fibers and is sus-

pended from the ciliary body. These ligaments can change the shape of the lens as tension is applied and released, so that the eye can focus on objects that are either nearby or far away. This process of adjustment is known as **accommodation**.

There are spaces between the cornea and

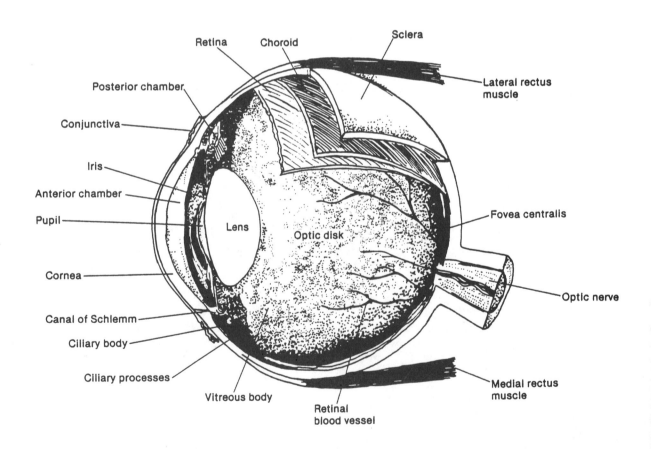

Figure 17: The eyeball, transverse section.

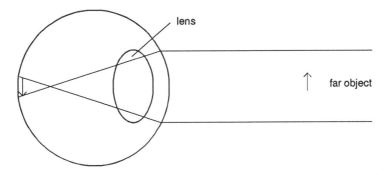

Light from distant objects are parallel when they reach the eye and can be focused without changes in lens.

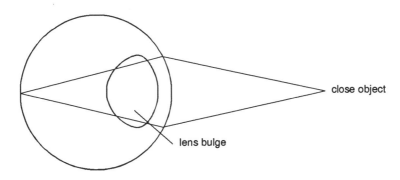

Light from close objects diverges and requires lens to bulge to focus object perfectly on the retina.

Figure 18: Focusing mechanism of the eye.

iris and between the iris and the lens. These chambers are filled with a fluid called **aqueous (AY-kwee-us) humor** that is formed in the ciliary body. It flows across the front of the eye, maintaining a constant pressure in the chambers. Finally, it is absorbed into the bloodstream through a network of tissue known as the **drainage angle**.

Behind the lens is the **vitreous (VIT-ree-us) body**, which is a space filled with a transparent jelly-like substance called **vitreous humor**. Its function is to maintain the shape of the eyeball and support the retina.

Rods and Cones. When light enters the eye through the cornea, iris, and lens, it is **refracted** (or bent) so that it can be **focused** onto the retina (see Figure 18). (Color is determined by the wavelength of the light.) The light forms an image on the retina and that image is inverted because of the bending of the light. The image is then converted into nerve impulses by the rods and cones, transmitted to ganglion cells by bipolar neurons, then sent to the cerebral cortex via the optic nerve to be interpreted and, acted upon if necessary. The brain receives two images, one from each eye. They are slightly different and must be blended to form a single, three-dimensional image. To achieve this, the two pictures must be on corresponding areas of the two retinas. This requires adjustments of the eyes. If these adjustments are not made, double vision occurs.

The rods and cones are named for their

different shapes and they also have a different chemical composition and different roles. The rods, which detect only black and white, are specialized for seeing in the dark. They contain a pigment called **rhodopsin (roh-DOP-sin)**, which is very sensitive to light. When lights strikes a rod, rhodopsin breaks down into its two components—**scotopsin (skoh-TOP-sin)** and a derivative of vitamin A called **retinene (RET-ih-neen)**. This chemical process generates nerve impulses. In bright light, the breakdown occurs so rapidly that the supply of rhodopsin cannot keep up with the demand. Lack of rhodopsin or visual purple leads to night blindness. Rhodopsin is obtained mainly from vitamin A.

The cones, in contrast, are designed to receive bright light and color. They contain a substance that is slightly different than rhodopsin and is sensitive to certain frequencies of light. This substance will not break down except in bright light and it reforms quickly. Individual cones specialize in a particular color—red, green, or blue. Other colors are combinations of these three, and all of them together appear as white.

The rods and cones adjust to the amount of light present by the supply of pigment they can maintain. In continuous bright light, even the cones eventually cannot keep up a supply of pigment and the eyes eventually become less sensitive. In continued darkness or dim light, the supply of pigment is plentiful and the eye is more able to react to any available light. These phenomena are known as **light and dark adaptation**.

HEARING AND BALANCE

The ear is an organ that is almost as complex as the eye (see Figure 19). It has two separate functions: It governs both the auditory sense and the sense of balance or position. Most of the structure of the ear is designed to hear sounds. Only the **semicircular (SEM-ee-SER-kyoo-lar) canals** and the **vestibule (VES-tih-byool)** in the inner ear are related to balance.

Structure

The ear consists of three sections: the **outer ear**, the **middle ear**, and the **inner ear**. As their names suggest, each subsequent section is located deeper in the interior of the skull than the preceding one.

Outer Ear. The outer ear consists of three components. The **pinna (PIN-nah)**, which we ordinarily call the ear, is the flap of skin and cartilage on the outside of the head. The **external auditory canal** extends from the pinna to about 4 cm into the skull, ending at the tympanic membrane. The **tympanic (tim-PAN-ick) membrane** or eardrum is a thin membrane with skin on the outside and mucous membrane on the inside that completely separates the outer ear from the middle ear. It is attached in such a way that it vibrates when struck by sound waves.

Middle Ear. The next section is the middle ear, a cavity in the temporal bone. It is full of air and is connected to the upper part of the throat (the nasopharynx) by a tube called the **auditory tube** or **eustachian (yoo-STAY-kee-an) tube**. Inside the middle ear are three bones called the **hammer (malleus (MAL-ee-us))**, **anvil (incus (ING-kus))**, and **stirrup (stapes (STAY-peez))** because of their shapes. These bones form a moveable chain between the eardrum and the oval window of the inner ear. When the eardrum vibrates, those bones amplify and pass the sound waves across the middle ear to the inner ear.

Inner Ear. The inner ear is also called the labyrinth. It has a bony outer shell and a membranous lining. There are three major structures in the inner ear: the vestibule, in the center, the semicircular canals above the vestibule, and the **cochlea (KOCK-lee-ah)** below the vestibule.

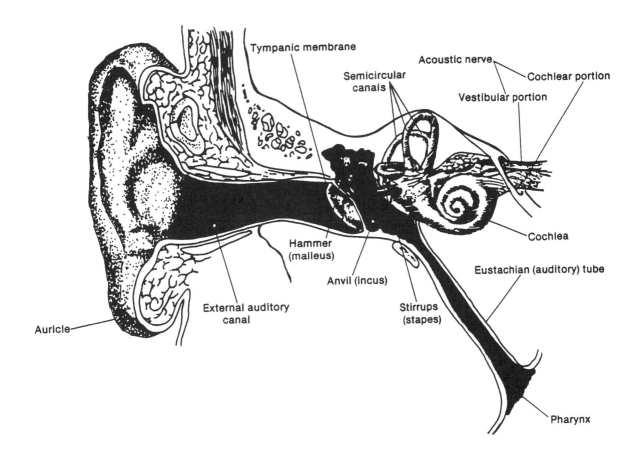

Figure 19: The ear.

They contain several fluid-filled sacs and tubes composed of the membranous lining. The sacs are surrounded by a fluid called **perilymph (PER-ih-limf)** and are filled with a slightly different fluid called **endolymph (END-doh-limf)**. The structures are the **cochlear (KOCK-lee-ar) duct** (tube in the cochlea), the **utricle (YOO-tree-kul)** and **saccule (SACK-yool)** (sacs in the vestibule), and the **semicircular ducts** (tubes in the semicircular canals).

The vestibule is a small chamber that is separated from the middle ear by an oval-shaped "window" of membrane. The stapes bone rests against this window and communicates sound waves to the fluid in the inner ear by vibrating against the window. A second window, the round window is located below the oval window and bends out as the stapes pushes the oval window in. This prevents ex-

cessive pressure in the inner ear. On the other side of the windows it the cochlea, which is spiral-shaped like a snail shell. Within the cochlea the floor of the duct is called the **basilar (BAS-ih-lar) membrane**, and the receptor for hearing—the **organ of Corti (KOR-tee)**—rests on it. This organ is made up of a ribbon-like arrangement of cells with tiny hairs. As the fluid in the cochlear duct moves, these hairs move with it and initiate sensory nerve impulses that represent sound. These impulses travel along the cochlear nerves to the auditory cortex in the cerebrum.

Sound

The number of times a sound wave vibrates per second is called its frequency and determines its pitch. For example, middle C on the musical scale is produced by sound waves vibrating at a frequency of 256 cycles per second (cps). [Cycles per second (cps) and hertz (Hz) are often used interchangeably in the discussion of sound frequencies.] The C an octave higher (C above middle C) is 512 cps. The human ear may be able to hear sounds ranging in frequency from 16 cps to 20,000 cps, but individuals vary in their hearing ability and the ability to hear high frequencies tends to decrease with age.

The loudness (volume) of a sound is determined by the height of the sound waves, which is measured in decibels (db). The human ear can detect sound volumes from 0 db (defined as the threshold of hearing) to about 120 to 140 db. After that, the ear will register pain rather than sound, and the ear may be damaged by exposure to such sounds.

Balance

Position or equilibrium is monitored by the vestibule and by the third structure in the inner ear, the semicircular canals. There are three of these canals or tubes arranged in semicircles. Each is positioned in a different geometric plane at right angles to the others. The canals are lined with semicircular ducts, which connect to the sac called the utricle in the vestibule. At the point where each duct connects to the sac, there is a widened area called an **ampulla (am-PUL-lah)**. Each ampulla has receptor cells on its walls, with hairs on the outside edge. These hairs are called the **cristae (KRIS-tee)**. Movements of the head cause the fluid in the semicircular ducts to move and stimulate the cristae. This generates nerve impulses that travel along the vestibular branches of the acoustic nerve to the cerebral cortex. The brain can use this information to send the necessary messages to the body to maintain balance during movement.

The floor of the utricle also has a patch of sensory cells called **maculae (MACK-yoo-lee)** that have hairs on them. Particles of calcium carbonate called **otoliths (OH-toh-lith)** float in the fluid that fills the inner ear. The otoliths move in response to the pull of gravity (inertia) and brush against the hairs of the maculae. The movement of the hairs stimulates a nerve impulse that carries information to the cerebral cortex.

STOP AND REVIEW

Short answers

1. Name the special senses.

   a. _____

   b. _____

   c. _____

   d. _____

   e. _____

2. Name the two locations for taste receptors.

    a. _____

    b. _____

3. Where are olfactory receptors located? _____

4. Name the two structures located at the corner of each eye closest to the nose.

    a. _____

    b. _____

Fill in the blanks

5. The eyeball is set in a cavity in the skull called the _____

6. The eyelids are lined with a membrane called the _____

7. The gland located at the upper outer edge of each eye is the _____

8. The receptors for vision are located in the _____

9. Rods are designed for _____ vision.

10. Rods contain pigment called _____

11. The cones are designed for _____ vision.

12. The rods and cones adjust to the amount of light present by the supply of _____ they maintain.

13. The two functions of the inner ear are _____ and _____

True or false

14. Most of the structure of the ear is designed for balance. T/F

DISORDERS AND DISEASES OF THE SENSE ORGANS

Disorders of Smell and Taste

Disorders of smell and taste are rare and usually related to damage to the olfactory nerve. Occasionally, a person will lose his or her sense of smell temporarily when nasal congestion interferes with the contact between odors and the olfactory receptors in the nose. The ability to detect odors almost always returns when the congestion is relieved. Another possible cause of **anosmia (an-OZ-mee-ah)** or loss of the sense of smell is **nasal polyps (POL-ips)**. Polyps are benign abnormal growths caused by overproduction of fluid by mucous membranes. Elderly persons may also gradually lose some of their ability to taste and smell; this may affect their interest in eating. Such patients should be urged to eat a good, balanced diet even if their enjoyment of food is reduced.

People who suffer head injuries often lose their sense of smell because the olfactory bulb has been torn on one or both sides. Patients who undergo craniotomy in the frontal area of the brain can also experience a loss of smell. This usually occurs when the olfactory nerves have been severed during removal of a tumor.

The eyes and ears, in contrast, are subject to a number of different disorders. First we will look at eye problems, then at disorders of the ear. Special instruments to examine, evaluate, and treat such problems are used in many physicians' offices (Table 7).

Table 7: Equipment Used to Diagnose and Treat Eye and Ear Disorders

Ophthalmoscope (of-THAL-moh-skohp)	A hand-held instrument with an intense, focused light that is used to look at the interior of the eye and focus on the retina.
Snellen Chart	A chart with letters of varying sizes printed on it, which is used to test a patient's vision.
Audiometer (AW-dee-OM-eh-ter)	A machine with earphones attached that emits measured sounds and includes a device for the patient to indicate when he or she hears the sound. The record of the patient's responses is called an audiogram.
Hearing Aid	There are several types of hearing aids. The behind-the-ear aid has a microphone, amplifier, and a battery that is worn behind the ear and is attached to an earphone (speaker) that is inserted into the ear. The bone conduction aid bypasses the middle ear and transmits sound waves through the skull by translating them into vibrations on the mastoid process, a bone just behind the ear. A body-worn aid is similar to the behind-the-ear aid, but the amplifier is larger and must be worn on the body.
Impedance (im-PEED-ans) Testing	In this procedure a probe is inserted into the ear and a seal obtained. The probe emits sounds and measures their reflection or rebound from the eardrum. This test is used to determine the flexibility of the eardrum.
Electrocochleography (ee-LECK-troh-KOCK-lee-OG-rah-fee)	This test measures electrical activity in the cochlea, using a probe that penetrates the eardrum.
Tonometer (toh-NOM-eh-ter)	When pressed against the anesthetized cornea this instrument measures intraocular pressure.

DISEASES AND DISORDERS OF THE EYE

Refraction Errors

Normally, the light that enters the eye is refracted by the cornea, lens, and other structures in the eye so that it focuses exactly on the retina. However, many people's eyes are slightly different from the norm, and this causes vision problems. Such problems may be present at birth or may develop later in life. As a person grows older, the eyes change and so does vision. The four most common problems of refraction are **myopia (mye-OH-pee-ah)**, **hypermetropia (HYE-per-meh-TROH-pee-ah)**, **presbyopia (PRES-bee-OH-pee-ah)**, and **astigmatism (ah-STIG-mah-tizm)**.

Myopia. In nearsightedness, the eye is too long from cornea to retina. Objects that are far away, therefore, are focused in front of the retina and do not form a clear image.

Hypermetropia. In farsightedness, the eye is too short from front to back. This means that objects close to the eye are focused behind the retina, and again the retina does not receive a clear image.

Presbyopia. As a person ages the lens tends to harden and lose flexibility. This condition, known as presbyopia, typically makes it difficult to focus on close objects. Convex reading glasses can help but can also cause distant objects to be out of focus. Bifocal lenses provide the ability to see both distant and close objects without removing the glasses. These lenses can also conform to any previous lens prescriptions.

Contact lenses are evolving from hard, impermeable lenses to the newer soft, gas-permeable lenses. Although the new lenses are more easily tolerated, they cannot correct for some of the conditions that hard lenses can.

Surgical procedures—such as **radial ker-atotomy (KER-ah-TOT-oh-mee)**, a radiating series of incisions on the cornea that reduces its curvature—may become more common in the future, providing an alternative to corrective lenses.

Astigmatism. This is distortion caused by uneven curvature of the cornea. The person with astigmatism may be able to get a clear image of vertical lines but not of horizontal lines, or the opposite may be true. This problem usually is present at birth and does not change with age.

All four of these problems can be corrected with glasses or (except for presbyopia) contact lenses. These devices provide an artificial lens that is ground specifically to compensate for the problem in the eye's structure. Glasses or lenses are prescribed by an **ophthalmologist (OF-thal-MOL-oh-jist)** or an **optometrist (op-TOM-eh-trist)** based on extensive tests of the patient's vision. The prescription is filled by an **optician (op-TISH-an)**. An ophthalmologist is a medical doctor who treats eye diseases and performs eye surgery in addition to testing patients for vision problems. An optometrist is trained specifically to test and prescribe for problems of refraction but is not a physician. An optician is trained to grind lenses and fit glasses and contacts according to a prescription supplied by an optometrist or an ophthalmologist.

INFECTION AND INFLAMMATION OF THE EYE

Sty

A **sty** is an infection of the follicle of an eyelash. It causes a painful, red swelling that develops a white center and eventually bursts, thus relieving the pain. Relief can be obtained by applying hot compresses to the inflamed area for 15 minutes several times a day. An antibiotic may also be prescribed to prevent the infection from spreading. In general, however, sties clear up by themselves within about a week.

Chalazion

A **chalazion (kah-LAY-zee-on)** is a small, painless lump on the edge of the eyelid caused by blockage of a gland in the eyelid. If it becomes infected, it will be red and painful. Large or infected chalazions should be treated by a doctor. The process may involve opening and draining the inflamed area. Otherwise, they usually last a month or two and may eventually go away without treatment.

Conjunctivitis

Conjunctivitis (kon-JUNK-tih-VYE-tis), or pink eye, is an inflammation of the conjunctiva caused by irritation, infection (baterial or viral) or by an allergic reation. The white of the eye turns red or pink, and there may be a discharge of pus that forms a crust overnight. Conjunctivitis may be contagious, so it is important for the problem to be treated with antibiotics if it is a bacterial infection. The patient should avoid touching the eye, keep his or her hands clean, and use a different towel and washcloth from other family members.

Corneal Ulcers and Infections

The cornea may be injured by a scratch, a blow, or by excessive wearing of non-gas permeable contact lenses. The wound may then become infected. The affected eye will be painful or at least uncomfortable, and the sclera will become reddened. An ulcer (erosion or defect) may be visible as a white spot or patch on the surface of the eye. Such an ulcer or infection can leave a scar on the cornea that may reduce vision. Also, if the problem is not treated it may spread to the interior of the eye and cause serious damage. Treatment is usually an ointment or drops chosen for the type of infection, which may be viral, fungal, or bacterial. Surgery may be necessary if the cornea is damaged, either to repair it or to replace it with a transplanted cornea.

Iritis

In this disorder, the tissue of the iris becomes inflamed. The ciliary body may also be involved. Cells from the inflamed area flake off and float in the aqueous humor in the chamber between the iris and cornea. These dead cells can interfere slightly with vision, if they are numerous. Also, the cells may stick to the cornea. The affected eye becomes red and painful or uncomfortable. If the problem is not treated, the cells may eventually block the opening through which aqueous humor drains out of the eye, causing acute **glaucoma (glaw-KOH-mah)**, which is discussed later in this chapter. **Iritis** is treated with ointment or eyedrops to reduce inflammation. The eye should also be checked regularly for any increase in pressure until the inflammation clears up. Iritis may return after the inflammation seems to be cured, but if it is treated it should eventually resolve completely and the patient's vision will return to normal.

Scleritis

This terms means inflammation of the sclera. It may occur by itself or along with rheumatoid arthritis or digestive tract disorders such as Crohn's disease. If it affects the back of the eye, vision may be impaired. In some cases, the tissue of the sclera is damaged. Steroid drugs, which reduce inflammation, are usually used to treat **scleritis (sklee-RYE-tis)**. In severe cases, immunosuppressive drugs may be prescribed to depress the inflammatory response. If tissue is damaged, surgical repair may be necessary.

STRUCTURAL DISORDERS OF THE EYE

Strabismus

Strabismus **(strah-BIZ-mus)** or crossed eyes are the result of malalignment by the muscles that control eye movement. In this disorder, the eyes do not focus on an object together. One of them stays still or moves in the opposite direction from the other. This problem may be present at birth or become apparent 3 months or more after birth as the baby learns to focus. It can also occur in adults. In children, the affected eye becomes "lazy" or **amblyopic (AM-blee-OH-pick)**—that is, it is no longer used and becomes progressively weaker. This occurs because a person will see a double image if the two eyes are used together without focusing and the brain compensates for this by ignoring the input from one eye. In children, strabismus is treated by putting a patch over the working eye, thus forcing the other to work and become stronger. Medication and glasses may be prescribed as well. If this treatment does not work, surgery to adjust the muscles may be necessary.

In adults, crossed eyes are caused by a disorder of the nerves or the muscles. Diabetes, hypertension, brain injury, and other diseases can cause this condition. The main symptom is double vision (diplopia). Treatment of the cause will usually resolve the problem in adults.

Entropion and Extropion

These terms mean in-turning (**entropion; en-TROH-pee-on**) and out-turning (**extropion; ecks-TROH-pee-on**) of the eyelashes. The edge of the lid, usually the lower lid, turns toward or away from the eyeball. In entropion, the eyelashes rub against the eye and may irritate the cornea and/or the conjunctiva. In extropion, part of the eye is overexposed and is not properly lubricated. This can lead to corneal ulcers. Both conditions occur most often in older people as a result of weakening of the muscles or fibrous tissue in the eyelids. They can also be caused by a scar on the face that distorts the tissue around the eye. The treatment for these problems is surgical repair of the weakened or distorted tissue.

Cataracts

A **cataract (KAT-ah-rack)** is a cloudy or opaque area in the lens of the eye. It may be caused by eye injuries or exposure to radiation or extreme heat or it may be inherited. Cataracts usually occur in both eyes, most commonly in older people. The opaque area may be so small that is has little effect at first, but it usually gradually enlarges until it affects the penetration of light into the eye, causing loss of vision and sometimes blurred vision. Vision can sometimes be helped by glasses, especially if only one eye is affected. In severe cases, the lens is removed surgically. This causes hypermetropia which can be corrected with contact lenses, glasses or a lens implant.

Color Blindness

Color blindness is the inability to detect certain colors. It is usually present at birth and is inherited. Almost all color blindness occurs in men because the ability to see color is a sex-linked genetic characteristic. Color blindness is due to the absence or deficiency of one type of cone on the retina. The most common form is the inability to tell reds from greens, especially in dim light. There is no treatment for color blindness.

Retinal Detachment

This condition is usually the result of a small hole in the retina that allows the retina to gradually pull away from the choroid. The vitreous humor seeps into the hole and works the retina loose, causing gradual loss of vision. Early symptoms of **retinal detachment** are flashes of light that may be seen by the patient just before the hole forms, and black, cobweb-like shapes that the patient may see as the hole is made. Areas of the peripheral vision may subsequently be lost. If the problem is discovered early, before the hole forms, the weak area of the retina can be repaired with a **laser** or a beam of intense, focused light. If the detachment has begun, the vitreous humor between the retina and choroid is removed so the retina can return to its normal location; the hole is then repaired.

Retinal Vessel Occlusion

The artery that supplies blood to the retina or the vein that drains it can become occluded (blocked) by a clot or embolism, either because of a clotting disorder or because of general circulatory problems. If the artery is blocked, the result is immediate full or partial blindness in that eye. If the vein is affected, vision is blurred. A blocked retinal artery requires immediate treatment to prevent permanent loss of vision. First, drugs are given to dissolve the clot and to prevent further clotting. If that does not work, surgery may be needed to remove the clot and restore blood flow.

If the problem occurs in a retinal vein, it may repair itself. The blood that leaks out of the occluded vein may be absorbed naturally. However, new veins may develop in various parts of the eye to compensate for the blockage, and these veins break easily and repeat the problem. If the leaked blood is not absorbed, permanent damage may be done to the eye. There is no useful treatment for this occlusion except control of any underlying disorder such as high blood pressure that may contribute to it.

Exophthalmos

This term means bulging of the eyes out of the orbits. It is caused by swelling of the tissue around and behind the eyeball as the result of one of several problems including **orbital cellulitis** (inflammation of the tissue behind the eye), **hyperthyroidism**, and a tumor behind the eye. The eye may become dry and may not be able to move freely, causing double vision. Treatment of the condition that is causing **exophthalmos (ECK-sof-THAL-mos)** may cure it, but in thyroid conditions additional treatment may be needed, such as suturing the lids together at the corners so that they cover more of the eye, steroid drugs to reduce inflammation, and occasionally an operation to reduce pressure behind the eye.

Glaucoma

There are two forms of glaucoma: **acute** or **angle-closure glaucoma** and **chronic** or **open-angle glaucoma**. The term glaucoma refers to a condition in which aqueous humor cannot drain normally out of the eye. Aqueous humor is constantly produced by the ciliary body, and it flows through the chambers on either side of the iris to a network of tissue called the drainage angle. From there it enters a drainage channel and is absorbed into a network of blood vessels. In glaucoma, the drainage angle and/or the channel become blocked. Pressure builds up in the chambers. Then, as the lens presses against the rest of the eye, pressure also builds up in the vitreous humor. This collapses the blood vessels on the retina, and the rods and cones, deprived of their needed blood supply, begin to die. The optic nerve may also be damaged. Vision quickly fades.

Acute glaucoma occurs when blockage of the drainage angle happens suddenly. In this case, the iris is pushed forward by an increase in the size of the lens due to aging. The outer edge of the iris blocks the drainage angle when the iris contracts to open the pupil in dim light. The symptoms begin with short periods of blurred vision and seeing haloes around lights. There may be pain and redness in the eye. Later, the attacks last longer and the pain becomes severe. If it is not treated, the optic nerve and rods and cones may be damaged and permanent loss of vision may occur. Treatment begins with reducing pressure in the eye by giving drops to make the pupil contract and diuretic drugs to reduce body fluids. Then, an operation called an **iridectomy (IR-ih-DECK-toh-mee)** is performed to make a new drainage channel through the iris. If acute glaucoma occurs in one eye, it is likely to occur in the other later, and the physician will want to check the patient's eyes regularly to monitor their internal pressure.

Chronic glaucoma occurs when blockage

of the drainage angle and the buildup of pressure in the eye happen slowly over a period of years. In early stages, it can only be detected by a special eye test to measure pressure in the eye. The disease progresses slowly if it is not detected, causing gradual loss of peripheral vision. At first, the other eye compensates and the patient may not notice the loss. If it is not treated, blindness results. Chronic glaucoma almost always affects both eyes, one after the other. Treatment for chronic glaucoma is the same as for acute glaucoma, except that drug treatment that reduces fluids may be sufficient and surgery is only necessary in severe cases.

DISORDERS OF THE EAR

Hearing loss can occur for two reasons: a failure of the mechanism that directs sound waves through the ear, which is known as **conductive hearing loss**, and damage to the nerves, which is called **sensorineural (SEN-soh-ree-NYOO-ral) hearing loss**. In the elderly, deafness may be caused by gradual deterioration of the cochlea and the auditory nerve. Exposure to loud noises for an extended time can cause the same sort of hearing loss as has been demonstrated in industrial workers and persons attending overamplified rock concerts. Sensorineural hearing loss cannot be reversed medically or surgically, although hearing can be improved by hearing aids in many cases. Most hearing problems in younger people are conductive and can be treated successfully.

Blockage of the Outer Ear
The two most common causes of blockage of the outer ear are wax buildup and infection. Glands in the outer ear produce a waxy substance called **cerumen (seh-ROO-men)** that lubricates the canal. Sometimes, an excessive amount of wax builds up in the ear and blocks it, causing hearing loss. When the wax is re-

moved, usually by putting warm water in the ear with a syringe and letting it run out again, hearing is restored.

Infections of the outer ear often occur after swimming in lakes and rivers where water may be polluted. The infection usually causes itching, then pain, and finally a greenish discharge. Some hearing loss may occur. The treatment consist of cleaning out the infected area and using a prescribed ointment or cream, either an antibiotic or a fungicide, occasionally combined with a steroid drug, depending on the type of organism that caused the infection.

Otitis Media
Otitis media (oh-TYE-tis MEE-dee-ah) means infection of the middle ear. It is usually a complication of a viral or bacterial infection in the nose or throat that has traveled up the eustachian tube. Otitis media is a common problem in children. The condition can be very painful. It may cause the eardrum to rupture, which eases the pain. This is more common with a bacterial infection than with a virus. Treatment usually consists of an antibiotic drug for bacterial infection, and a **myringotomy (MIR-in-GOT-oh-mee)** or lancing of the eardrum if it is bulging out. (Tubes may be inserted in the eardrum to relieve pressure, but they require special care.) The eardrum heals in a few weeks. If the condition is caused by a virus, treatment is usually not necessary and the infection subsides in about a week.

A chronic form of otitis media may occur because of a persistent bacterial infection. Such an infection may not cause any symptoms except an occasional discharge from the ear, hearing loss from a hole in the eardrum, and possible damage to the malleus, incus, or stapes. It can also spread to the bone behind the ear. **Cholesteatoma (KOH-leh-STEE-ah-TOH-mah)** is a particularly serious form of the disorder. The eustachian tube becomes blocked, and a ball of dead cells builds up against the eardrum. The ball becomes infected and the infection damages the delicate bones in the middle ear. The infection can then spread to the surrounding bone and even to the brain.

Persistent or severe infections are treated with antibiotics and by surgically cleaning out the affected area of the ear. In some cases, the mastoid bone must be removed or the structures inside the ear must be repaired or removed.

Otosclerosis

In **otosclerosis (OH-toh-sklee-ROH-sis)** abnormal bone cells grow between the vestibule of the inner ear and the stapes in the middle ear. The stapes gradually becomes immobilized and is less able to rock in the oval window and pass sound waves on to the nervous system. The disease may progress rapidly or slowly and may affect one or both ears. The current treatment is an operation called a **stapedectomy (STAY-peh-DECK-toh-mee)** in which the surgeon replaces the rigid, "frozen" stapes with a mobile substitute. This operation is not always successful, so it should only be performed on one ear at a time.

Ruptured Eardrum

The eardrum may rupture as the result of an infection, an explosion, a blow to the head, or an attempt to clean the ear with a sharp object. Rupture causes slight pain, possibly some hearing loss, and sometimes a discharge of either blood or pus. The eardrum usually heals itself and should be kept dry. Some physicians may prescribe an antibiotic to clear up any infection present or to prevent infection. If it does not heal, a number of procedures can be used to speed up the progress. There is usually no lasting damage to the hearing.

Cerebrospinal Fluid Otorrhea

Cerebrospinal fluid leaking through the ear canal (usually from a fracture of the skull base or a complication of ear surgery) can cause meningitis or brain abscess. Bruising behind the ear can indicate a basilar skull fracture, and clear fluid will drip from the ear canal, leaving a "halo" on the patient's pillow.

DISORDERS OF BALANCE

There are two major disorders of balance: Meniere's disease and labyrinthitis. An acoustic neuroma may also cause this condition.

Meniere's Disease

Meniere's (MEN-ee-AYRZ) disease is most commonly found in men between the ages of 40 and 60. In 90% of all cases, it is found in one ear only. The cause of this rare disorder is unknown. Excess fluid forms in the semicircular canals of the ear, putting extra pressure on the membranous structures of the canals, the vestibule, and also the cochlea. This membrane may rupture, disturbing the sense of balance. The symptoms are occasional attacks of dizziness that vary in frequency and last from a few hours to several days. Hearing loss, nausea and vomiting, or a feeling of pressure and ringing in the ear may also occur. Severe cases can cause anxiety because the patient cannot predict when an attack will come and he or she will suddenly lose equilibrium. Diagnosis is made by a series of hearing tests with the patient taking a diuretic drug between tests. The diuretic will reduce the pressure in the ear and cause an improvement in the patient's hearing if he or she has Meniere's disease. Other tests, including electrocochleography may be needed to make a definite diagnosis. Treatment may include **antivertiginous (AN-tih-ver-TIJ-ih-nus)** drugs, diuretic drugs, or, if the case is severe, an operation in which the surgeon creates a drain for the fluid that carries it into the cerebrospinal fluid. In debilitating cases, the semicircular canals may have to be destroyed.

Labyrinthitis

The labyrinth is another name for the inner ear. In this disorder, the membrane inside the inner ear becomes inflamed, usually due to a virus. The structure can no longer function properly, and severe dizziness occurs. Also, the eyes move slowly one way, then flick back the other way. This is called **nystagmus (nis-TAG-mus)**.

Nausea and vomiting may accompany the dizziness. **Labyrinthitis (LAB-ih-rin-THYE-tis)** usually clears within 6 weeks. The physician may prescribe an antianxiety drug to relax the patient, a vestibular depressant, and antiemetics for nausea. The patient may be advised to stay in bed for a few days until the worst of the symptoms are gone.

In the rare instance of bacterial labyrinthitis, the affected ear is completely destroyed and hearing is totally absent. This is a warning to observe closely for the development of meningitis or brain abscess.

Acoustic Neuroma

This condition is characterized by a benign tumor involving the eighth cranial nerve. Symptoms include unilateral hearing loss and various other complications depending on the size of the tumor. Neurosurgery is performed to remove the tumor, but such surgery does not restore hearing.

STOP AND REVIEW

Matching

Match the equipment listed with the eye and ear disorders it is used to diagnose or treat.

Equipment

a. ___ electrocochleography

b. ___ audiometer

c. ___ Snellen chart

d. ___ ophthalmoscope

e. ___ impedance testing

Disorders

1. A hand-held instrument with an intense, focused light that is used to look at the interior of the eye and focus on the retina

2. Measures electrical activity in the cochlea using a probe that penetrates the eardrum

3. Printed letters of varying sizes that are used to test a patient's vision

4. A machine with earphones attached that emits measured sounds and includes a device for the patient to indicate when he/she hears the sound.

5. A probe is inserted into the ear and a seal obtained. The probe emits sounds and measures their reflection or rebound from the eardrum. The test is used to determine the flexibility of the eardrum.

Match the eye condition with its definition.

Infection/Inflammation

a. ___ iritis

b. ___ scleritis

c. ___ corneal ulcers and infections

d. ___ conjunctivitis

e. ___ chalazion

f. ___ sty

Definition

1. A small, painless lump on the edge of the eyelid caused by blockage of a gland in the eyelid

2. An infection of the hair follicles of an eyelash

3. Occurs when the wound caused by an injury to the cornea resulting from a scratch or a blow becomes infected

4. An inflammation of the tissue of the iris

5. An inflammation of the conjunctiva caused by irritation, infection, or an allergic reaction

6. An inflammation of the sclera that can occur by itself or along with rheumatoid arthritis or digestive tract disorders.

A

Abdominal reflex Reflex (drawing in of the abdominal wall) elicited by stroking the side of the abdomen.

Abducens nerve Cranial nerve (VI) responsible for eye movement.

Accommodation Adjustment that allows the eye to focus at various distances.

Acetylcholine (ACh) An excitatory neurotransmitter.

Achilles reflex Ankle-jerk reflex elicited by tapping the Achilles tendon in the ankle.

Acoustic neuroma Benign tumor of the eighth cranial nerve.

Action potential Progress of a stimulus along the neuron.

Acupuncture Puncturing the body along specific meridian points with needles; used to block pain.

Adequate stimulus Stimulus that is sufficient to initiate a nerve impulse.

Afferent neurons Nerve cells that carry messages to the central nervous system from the peripheral nervous system.

Afferent nerve pathways Part of the peripheral nervous system that transmits data in the form of sensations to the central nervous system.

Alzheimer's disease Death of the nerve cells of the frontal and temporal lobes of the cerebrum; usually of unknown origin, beginning in middle age; also known as presenile senile dementia.

Amblyopic eye "Lazy" eye that becomes progressively weaker as it is used less and less.

Amnesia Pathologic loss of memory.

Amphetamines Commonly abused CNS stimulants prescribed for weight loss.

Ampulla Widened area at the point where each semicircular duct connects to the utricle.

Amyotrophic lateral sclerosis Condition in which motor neurons die for no known reason, resulting in atrophy of the muscles, weakness, spasticity, and eventually overactivity of the reflexes and loss of motor control.

Analgesic A substance that blocks the sense of pain without causing unconsciousness.

Aneurysm A sac formed by the localized dilation of the wall of an artery, vein, or the heart.

Angiography A diagnostic technique in which a radiopaque contrast medium is injected into an artery through a catheter; the vessels are observed through x-rays or films.

Angiotensin Neurotransmitter that is also a hormone.

Anosmia Loss of the sense of smell.

Anterior median fissure See Ventral median fissure.

Anterior root See Ventral root.

Anterior spinothalamic pathway Pathway by which crude touch and pressure information travel up the spinal cord to the thalamus.

Antianxiety drugs Commonly abused medications that are prescribed to treat anxiety.

Antibiotics Medications that treat bacterial infections.

Anticoagulants Medications that help prevent abnormal clot formation.

Anticonvulsants Medications that prevent convulsions or seizures.

Antidiuretic hormone (ADH) Posterior pituitary hormone that regulates fluid balance by regulating kidney functions.

Antiemetics Medications that prevent or relieve nausea and vomiting.

Antihistamines Medications that help reduce inflammation in allergic reactions.

Antiparkinsonian drugs Medications that are used to treat Parkinson's disease.

Antipyretics Medications that reduce fever.

Antivertiginous drugs Medications that are used to treat vertigo (sensation of movement).

Anvil See Incus.

Aphasia Inability to speak, write, or comprehend written or spoken language; caused by damage to the cerebral cortex.

Apraxia Inability to carry out familiar, purposeful actions; especially impairment of the ability to use objects correctly.

Aqueous humor Fluid that forms in the ciliary body and fills various chambers of the eye.

Arachnoid Middle layer of the meninges, which cover the brain and spinal cord.

Ascending tracts Tracts of nerves in the spinal column that carry nerve impulses from the rest of the body to the brain.

Aspartic acid An excitatory neurotransmitter.

Association areas Areas of the cerebral cortex that integrate input and responses.

Astigmatism A distortion caused by uneven curvature of the cornea or lens; the light ray is not sharply focused on the retina.

Astrocytes Star-shaped neuroglial cells containing a central body and many fibrous projections; found in the brain and spinal cord; probably have a role in supplying blood to the central nervous system neurons.

Ataxia Inability to control voluntary muscle movements; may be caused by damage to the cerebellum or the motor area of the cerebral cortex.

Atheroma An abnormal, fibrous-covered, fatty mass within the artery.

Atherosclerosis A form of arteriosclerosis in which deposits of cholesterol and other lipid substances (atheromas) are formed in the arteries.

Audiometer Machine with earphones that emits measured sounds to test hearing.

Auditory area Area of the cerebral cortex that controls hearing.

Auditory tube See Eustachian tubes.

Aura Warning signals that occur before a migraine, such as irritability, nausea, and visual disturbances.

Autonomic nervous system Part of the peripheral nervous system that carries unconscious, involuntary messages to the smooth internal organs, to the heart muscle, and to endocrine and other glands. It is divided into the sympathetic and parasympathetic divisions.

Axon A cell projection; carries nerve impulses away from the nerve cell body; it branches at its termination, forming many synapses at other nerve cells or effector organs.

Axon hillock The site at which the axon is attached to its nerve cell body.

B

Babinski reflex Reflex (toe flexion) elicited by stroking the outside of the sole of the foot with a blunt object.

Babinski sign Extension of the big toe and fanning of the other toes on testing for Babinski reflex.

Barbiturates Commonly abused, sedative-hypnotic drugs.

Basal ganglia Masses of gray

matter with a network of nerve tracts in the cerebral cortex.

Basilar membrane Floor of the cochlear duct.

Bell's palsy A disorder in which the facial nerve on one side swells for no known reason or becomes pinched due to a tumor pressing on the nerve; causes paralysis of the facial muscles usually on one side.

Bipolar neuron Neuron which has one dendrite and one axon; the least numerous type of neuron.

Blood-brain barrier Mechanism that regulates which materials in the bloodstream can enter the brain.

Brachial plexus Network of small nerves that serve the brachial (arm) area.

Brain stem Stemlike part of the brain connecting the cerebral hemispheres to the spinal cord; composed of the pons, the medulla oblongata, and the midbrain.

C

CT scan See Computerized axial tomography.

CVA See Cerebrovascular accident.

Carotid arteriogram Angiogram that outlines the carotid arteries in the neck and the anterior and middle cerebral arteries of the brain.

Carpal tunnel A passageway between the carpal bones of the wrist and the ventral ligaments; nerves pass through this tunnel on their way from the brain to the hand.

Carpal tunnel syndrome Swelling of the tissue in the carpal tunnel from accumulated fluid, causing pressure at the median nerve accompanied by pain and burning or tingling in the fingers and hand.

Cataract A cloudy or opaque area in the lens of the eye or its capsule; usually occuring in both eyes; most common in the elderly.

Cell body Part of neuron which

holds the nucleus.

Cauda equina Nerve roots at the end of the spinal cord that extend below it like a horse's tail.

Central canal Open space that runs through the center of the spinal cord.

Central nervous system (CNS) One of the two major divisions of the nervous system; includes the brain and the spinal cord.

Central nervous system depressants Drugs that slow CNS activity.

Central nervous system stimulants Drugs that accelerate CNS activity.

Cerebellum The part of the brain that coordinates muscle movement, maintains muscle tone, balance and posture; situated at the back of the brain stem.

Cerebral cortex Convoluted layer of gray matter covering the cerebral hemispheres; governs thought, reasoning, memory, sensation, and voluntary movement.

Cerebral hemispheres Two halves of the main portions of the brain.

Cerebral hemorrhage Bleeding from a damaged blood vessel into brain tissue.

Cerebral nuclei Ganglia that are joined to each other, to the cerebral cortex, and to the spinal cord.

Cerebral palsy Brain damage that occurs during fetal development, during birth, or in early childhood; may affect mobility of limbs, muscle movements, hearing, vision, speech, etc.

Cerebrospinal fluid Fluid found within the subarachnoid space, the central canal of the spinal cord, and the four ventricles of the brain.

Cerebrospinal fluid otorrhea Leakage of cerebrospinal fluid through the ear canal, usually from a skull fracture.

Cerebrovascular accident Commonly called a stroke; caused by interruption of blood circulation to the brain resulting in tissue death; the severity depends on how much and what part of the brain is damaged.

Cerebrum Largest part of the brain; its two cerebral hemispheres are united by the corpus callosum.

Cerumen Waxy substance produced by glands in the outer ear; ear wax.

Cervical enlargement Enlargement at the top of the spinal cord.

Cervical nerves Eight pairs of spinal nerves that emerge between the cervical vertebrae.

Cervical plexus Network of small nerves that serve the cerevical (neck) area.

Cervical spondylosis Abnormal immobility and consolidation of the vertebrae in the neck.

Chalazion A small painless lump or mass on the edge of the eyelid, resulting from chronic inflammation of a gland in the eyelid.

Cholecystokinin Neurotransmitter that is also a hormone.

Cholesteatoma A serious form of otitis media in which the eustachian tube becomes blocked and a ball of dead cells or a cyst-like mass builds up in the eardrum.

Chorea Ceaseless, rapid, uncontrollable, jerky movements.

Choroid layer Thin vascular coat of the eye.

Choroid plexuses Networks of blood vessels in the ventricles of the brain.

Chronic fatigue syndrome A neuropsychological disorder which may be related to Epstein-Barr virus infection.

Chronic organic brain syndrome Broad range of senile dementia (decreased intellectual ability) in older adults.

Ciliary muscle Muscle that controls lens curvature to adjust vision.

Circle of Willis The circle of vessels near the base of the brain that supplies the brain with oxygen and nutrients.

Coccygeal nerve Nerve from which stems the last two spinal nerves.

Cochlea Spiral-shaped structure resembling a snail shell, that forms part of the inner ear.

Cochlear duct Spiral-shaped membranous tube within the cochlea.

Color blindness The inability to distinguish between certain colors; it is usually inherited by males through the mother; the most common form is red-green confusion.

Coma Unconsciousness from which the patient cannot be awakened, even by powerful stimuli.

Commissure A bridge of gray matter that joins the two portions of the spinal cord.

Computerized tomography (CT scan) A radiologic imaging method that produces a series of pictures of cross-sections of the brain and puts them together with a computer.

Concussion Loss of consciousness, transient or prolonged, resulting from a violent shock, jar, or blow to the head.

Conductive hearing loss Hearing loss caused by failure of the mechanism that directs sound waves through the ear.

Conductivity In neurology, the ability to transmit a stimulus such as a nerve impulse.

Cones Specialized cells in the retina that are sensitive to light.

Conjunctiva Mucous membrane that lines the eyelids.

Conjunctivitis An inflammation of the conjunctiva caused by bacterial or viral infection or allergic, chemical, or physical factors.

Contusion In neurology, bruising of brain tissue, causing loss of consciousness; often related to skull fractures.

Conus medullaris Bottom of the spinal cord where it tapers to a point.

Contralateral reflex Reflex in which the neurons cross from one side of the spinal cord to the other.

Cornea Transparent structure that forms the front of the eyeball.

Corneal reflex Reflex (eye closure) elicited by touching the cornea.

Corneal ulcer A white spot or patch on the surface of the eye's anterior covering; caused by an infection resulting from a scratch or blow.

Corpus callosum A mass of transverse white fibers that bridges the longitudinal fissure between the two cerebral hemispheres, providing a means of communication between the two hemispheres.

Costae Ribs.

Cranial sinuses Blood-filled spaces between the layers of dura

Cristae Hairs on the outside edge of the ampulla.

D

Delta waves Abnormal EEG wave.

Dendrite Thread-like extensions of the cytoplasm of a neuron; compose most of the receptive surface of a neuron.

Depolarization Reversal of the resting potential in nerve cells.

Dermatome Specific area of skin that is innervated by a particular spinal nerve.

Descending tracts Tracts of nerves in the spinal cord that carry nerve impulses from the brain to the rest of the body.

Diencephalon Posterior part of the forebrain, consisting of the thalamus and hypothalamus.

Disorientation Form of mental confusion in which the person does not know where he or she is or cannot identify the year or time of day.

Dopamine An inhibitory neurotransmitter.

Dorsal median sulcus Shallow groove on the posterior side of the spinal cord that divides it in half lengthwise.

Dorsal ramus (plural, rami) Branch of the spinal nerve.

Dorsal root Posterior root that attaches each spinal nerve to the spinal cord.

Dorsal root ganglion Swelling on the dorsal root that holds the cell bodies of sensory (afferent) neurons.

Drainage angle Network of tissue that absorbs aqueous humor and transfers it to the bloodstream.

Dura mater Outermost layer of the meninges, which cover the brain and spinal cord.

E

EEG See Electroencephalography.

Efferent nerve pathways Part of the peripheral nervous system that stimulates action, movement, or change.

Efferent neurons Nerve cells that carry impulses from the central nervous system to the peripheral nervous system; for example, a motor nerve.

Effector A muscle or a gland that performs a characteristic action when stimulated.

Electrocochleography Measurement of electrical activity in the cochlea, using a probe that penetrates the eardrum.

Electroencephalography A technique used for measuring the electrical activity of the brain; electrodes are attached to the skull and to a recording device that makes a tracing of the brain waves in the form of a graph.

Embolus (pl. emoboli) A blood clot or other piece of material travelling in the circulation from larger to smaller vessels, thus obstructing circulation.

Encephalitis An inflammation of brain tissue, usually due to viral infection.

Encephalon All portions of the brain considered together.

Endolymph Fluid that fills the sacs of the inner ear.

Endorphins Neurotransmitters that inhibit pain impulses.

Engrams Memories/learned behavior stored in association areas of the cerebral cortex.

Enkephalins Neurotransmitters that inhibit pain impulses.

Entropion In-turning of the eyelashes.

Ependymal cells Cells that form the inner lining of the cavities in the brain and of the central canal in the spinal cord.

Epidural abscess A pocket of infection marked by the collection of pus, situated upon or outside the dura mater; can result from bacterial invasion through small wounds or breaks in the skin.

Epilepsy Transient disturbances of the electrical activity of the brain that cause periodic seizures or spasms.

Epstein-Barr virus (EBV) infection An infection that causes infectious mononucleosis and may be linked to other infectious diseases.

Ethmoid bone Cranial bone that lies between the eye sockets.

Eustachian tube Channel from the tympanic cavity to the naso-pharynx; it adjusts the pressure in the cavity to the external air pressure.

Evoked response Stimulation of a specific part of the nervous system.

Excitability Readiness to respond to a stimulus; irritability.

Exophthalmos Abnormal protrusion or bulging of the eyes out of the orbit, caused by swelling of the tissue around and behind the eyeball, usually due to hyperthyroidism.

External auditory canal Portion of the outer ear that extends from the pinna to the tympanic mem-brane.

Exteroceptors A sensory nerve ending found in the skin; stimu-lated by the external environment and mucous membranes.

Extradural space Space between the dura mater and the vertebrae.

Extrapyramidal pathway Pathway by which voluntary muscle movements travel from the motor cortex to the spinal cord and then to the effector.

Extropion Out-turning of the eyelashes.

F

Facial nerve Cranial nerve (VII) responsible for taste, facial expression, and secretion of tears and saliva.

Fight or flight syndrome Automatic reactions to stress, such as increased heart rate, pupil dilation, and increased blood pressure.

Fit See Seizures.

Focus Convergence of light rays on the retina.

Friedreich's ataxia An inherited disease of the spinal column, affecting children, which causes degeneration of nerve fibers, resulting in a variety of symptoms.

Frontal bone Cranial bone in the forehead.

Funiculi Columns of white matter in the spinal cord.

G

Gamma-aminobutyric acid (GABA) An inhibitory neuro-transmitter.

Ganglion (pl. ganglia) A knot or knot-like mass; a group of nerve cell bodies located outside the central nervous system.

General sensory area Area of the cerebral cortex that controls discrimination of sensations.

Glaucoma A condition in which the aqueous humor cannot drain normally out of the eye increasing intraocular pressure; the two forms are acute (angle-closure) glaucoma and chronic (open-angle) glaucoma.

Glossopharyngeal nerve Cranial nerve (IX) responsible for taste, swallowing, and saliva excretion

Glutamic acid An excitatory neurotransmitter.

Glycine An inhibitory neurotransmitter.

Gray matter Bundles of unmyelinated nerve fibers, which appear gray because of the color of these fibers.

Guillain-Barré syndrome A form of peripheral neuropathy affecting especially the spinal nerves, but also the cranial nerves; symptoms appear suddenly; usually occurs as a complication of a viral infection or after immunization for a viral illness.

Gustatory area Area of the cerebral cortex that receives flavor sensations.

Gustatory cells Cells in the taste buds, which have microscopic hairs.

Gustatory sensors The receptors for taste, located mostly on the tongue, but also on the soft palate and in the throat.

H

Hammer See Malleus.

Hearing aid Device that amplifies sound to compensate for hearing loss.

Hemiplegia Paralysis of one side of the body, usually caused by a brain lesion, such as a tumor, or by a cerebral vascular accident.

Herpes zoster Disease caused by the chicken pox virus that results in inflammation of the spinal ganglia.

Histamine An excitatory neurotransmitter.

Homeostasis A steady state; the tendency of biological systems to maintain stability while continually adjusting to conditions optimal for survival.

Hormone-releasing factors Substances secreted by the

hypothalamus that signal the anterior pituitary gland to release its hormones.

Horns Legs of the "H" of gray matter in a cross-section of the spinal cord.

Huntington's chorea A rare, inherited disease, usually beginning in middle age, resulting from degenerative changes in the cerebral cortex and basal ganglia.

Hydrocephalus Enlargement of the head caused by excessive CSF.

Hypermetropia Farsightedness; visual defect in which parallel light rays focus behind the retina.

Hyperthyroidism Excess activity of the thyroid gland.

Hypoglossal nerve Cranial nerve (XII) responsible for tongue movement.

Hypothalamus Portion of the diencephalon, which regulates the pituitary gland.

I

Impedance testing Test of the opposition to the passage of sound waves by measuring the flexibility of the eardrum.

Incus Tiny anvil-shaped bone in the middle ear.

Inferior oblique muscle Muscle that rotates the eyeball upward and outward.

Inferior rectus muscle Muscle that rotates the eyeball downward and medially.

Inner ear Portion of the ear from the oval window to the cochlea.

Insula Section of the cerebral cortex inside the lateral fissure.

Intercostal nerves See Thoracic nerves.

Interneurons Neurons that form a bridge between primary afferent sensory neurons and final motor neurons; located in the brain and spinal cord. Also, any neuron whose processes lie entirely within a specific area, such as the olfactory lobe.

Iridectomy Surgical removal of

part of the iris.

Iris Circular pigmented structure behind the cornea.

Iritis A disorder in which the tissue of the iris becomes inflamed; the ciliary body may also be involved.

L

Labyrinth See inner ear.

Labyrinthitis A disorder in which the membrane inside the inner ear becomes inflamed, usually due to a virus; dizziness results.

Lacrimal duct Structure that leads to the lacrimal sac.

Lacrimal glands Glands located on the upper outer edge of each eye; they secrete tears, which keep the surface of the eye moist and clean.

Lacrimal sac Structure at the inner corner of the eye, which collects tears and drains into the nasal passages.

Laser Beam of intense, focused light that can be used for some types of surgery.

Lateral rectus muscle Muscle that abducts the eyeball.

Lateral spinothalamic pathway Pathway by which pain and temperature information travel up the spinal cord to the thalamus.

Lens Transparent body of the eye that aids in refraction.

Light and dark adaptation Ability of the eyes to adjust to any available light by varying the pigment supply in the rods and cones.

Limbic cortex Part of the cerebral cortex; believed to contain memories of past experiences; also called the emotional brain or the visceral brain.

Longitudinal fissure Deep fold in the cerebral cortex that divides it into two halves.

Lou Gehrig's disease See Amyotrophic lateral sclerosis.

Lumbar enlargement Enlargement at the bottom of the

spinal cord.

Lumbar nerve   Five pairs of spinal nerves that emerge between the lumbar vertebrae.

Lumbar plexus   Network of small nerves that serve the lumbar (low back) area.

Lumbar puncture · A diagnostic procedure in which a needle is inserted into the subarachnoid space between the third and fourth lumbar vertebrae and cerebrospinal fluid is removed; also called a spinal puncture.

Lyme disease   A bacterial disease carried by ticks.

M

Maculae   Patch of sensory cells on the floor of the utricle.

Malleus   Tiny hammer-shaped bone in the middle ear.

Mechanoreceptor   Receptor stimulated by mechanical pressure or distortion, as from touch and sound.

Medial rectus muscle   Muscle that adducts the eyeball.

Medulla oblongata   The lowest part of the brain stem, the base of the brain, a continuation of the spinal column with the pons above it; contains tracts of white matter that are the channels of communication between the spinal cord and the brain and nerve centers for both motor and sensory functions.

Memory traces   See Engrams.

Meniere's diseas   A rare disorder in which excess fluid forms in the semicircular canals, the vestibule, and the cochlea of the ear.

Meninges   Three layers of tissue that cover the brain and spinal cord.

Meningitis   Inflammation of the meninges; often occurs as a complication of a viral illness.

Methaqualone   Commonly abused hypnotic drug.

Microglia   Small non-neural cells found in the brain; when the brain tissue is inflamed or damaged, they grow larger. Their function is to clean debris and waste products in the brain; they are migratory.

Microsurgery   Surgery performed under a microscope to see tiny structures as they are repaired.

Midbrain   A short section of nerve tissue above the pons; contains nerve pathways between the cerebral hemispheres and the medulla oblongata.

Middle ear   Portion of the ear from the tympanic membrane to the oval window of the inner ear.

Migraine   Periodic, debilitating headaches; may be accompanied by nausea, vomiting or blurred vision, often limited to one side of the head.

Minor tranquilizer   Commonly abused drugs such as diazepam (Valium).

Mixed nerves   Nerves that contain sensory and motor neurons; spinal nerves.

Monosynaptic reflex   A simple reflex requiring only two neurons: one receptor and one effector.

Mood swings   Sudden changes in mood.

Motor nerve pathways   See Efferent nerve pathways.

Motor neuron   Neuron that transmits impulses from the central nervous system to the muscles and glands; an efferent neuron conveying motor impulses.

Motor speech area   Area of the cerebral cortex that controls formation of written and spoken words.

Motor tracts   See Descending tracts.

Multiple sclerosis (MS)   A chronic neurologic disease in which the white matter and occasionally the gray matter of the central nervous system has patches of demyelination. The disease primarily affects the myelin and not the nerve cells themselves; causes a number of different symptoms depending on which nerves are affected.

Multipolar neuron   Neuron that has a single axon and several dendrites; most are located in the central nervous system.

Myelin sheath   A layer of lipid substance wrapped around the axons of certain nerve fibers.

Myelography   A procedure used to visualize the interior of the spinal cord, in which a radiopaque substance is injected into the subarachnoid space of the spinal canal.

Myopia   Nearsightedness; visual defect in which the parallel light waves entering the eye are focused in front of the retina; a result of the eyeball being too long from front to back.

Myringotomy   Lancing of the eardrum, sometimes used to treat otitis media.

N

NREM   See Nonrapid eye movement sleep.

Nasal epithelium   Mucous lining of the upper part of the nasal passages.

Nasal polyps   Benign abnormal growths in the nose caused by overproduction of fluid by mucous membranes.

Nerve   Bundle of axons in the PNS.

Nerve fibers   See Axon.

Nerve impulses   Messages carried by nerves from one part of the body to another.

Nerve tracts   Bundle of axons in the CNS.

Neurilemma   Also spelled neurolemma; the plasma membrane of a Schwann cell forming sheath of Schwann of a myelinated or unmyelinated peripheral nerve.

Neurofibril nodes   See Nodes of Ranvier.

Neurofibrils   The delicate threads running through the cytoplasm of a nerve cell, extending into the axon and dendrites.

Neuroglia   Cells that provide the support functions of the nervous system; in the central nervous system, these are the astrocytes, oligodendroglia, and microglia.

Neuroglial cells See Neuroglia.

Neurons Nerve cells that carry nerve impulses to, from, and within the central nervous system; the working cells of the nervous system. Consists of a cell body containing a nucleus and its surrounding cytoplasm, the axon, and dendrites.

Neurotensin Neurotransmitter that is also a hormone.

Neurotransmitter A chemical substance that is released from the axon terminal of a presynaptic neuron on excitation and that travels across the synaptic cleft to either excite or inhibit the target cell; there are more than 40 different neurotransmitter chemicals supplying the brain.

Nociceptor Receptor stimulated by pain or injury.

Nodes of Ranvier Gaps at regular intervals in the myelin sheath along the axon so that the axon is enclosed only by Schwann cell processes.

Nonrapid eye movement sleep (NREM) A level of sleep, composed of four stages, which can be identified by EEG recordings of brain waves. NREM sleep is increased after physical activity.

Norepinephrine An excitatory neurotransmitter.

Nystagmus Rapid, involuntary movement of the eyeball.

O

Occipital bone Cranial bone that forms part of the posterior and inferior skull.

Oculomotor nerve Cranial nerve (III) responsible for eyeball and eyelid movement, regulation of pupil size, and accommodation for close vision.

Olfactory area Area of the cerebral cortex that receives odors.

Olfactory hairs Dendrites of sensory neurons in olfactory cells.

Olfactory nerve Cranial nerve (I) responsible for the sense of smell

Olfactory sensors The receptors for smell, found in the mucous lining of the upper part of the nose.

Oligodendrocytes A type of neuroglial cell that surrounds nerve cell bodies and their extensions and holds them together in bundles; also forms the myelin sheath in the central nervous system.

Ophthalmologist Medical doctor who treats eye diseases, performs eye surgery, and tests vision.

Ophthalmoscope Hand-held instrument with an intense, focused light, used to look at the interior of the eye and focus on the retina.

Optic nerve Cranial nerve (II) responsible for vision.

Optician Professional trained to grind lenses and fit contacts and glasses according to a prescription.

Optometrist Eye care professional trained to test and prescribe for refraction problems.

Orbit Cavity in the skull that holds the eye.

Orbital cellulitis Inflammation of the tissue behind the eye.

Organ of Corti Receptor for hearing composed of a ribbon-like arrangement of cells with tiny hairs.

Otitis media An infection of the middle ear; usually a complication of a viral or bacterial infection in the nose or throat; a common problem in infants and young children.

Otoliths Particles of calcium carbonate that float in inner ear fluid move in response to gravity.

Otosclerosis A disorder in which abnormal bone cells grow between the vestibule of the inner ear and the stapes in the middle ear.

Outer ear Portion of the ear that includes the pinna, external auditory and canal, and tympanic membrane.

Oxytocin Posterior pituitary hormone that stimulates uterine contractions during childbirth.

P

Palpebrae Protective cushions of skin that move up and down in front of the eyeball; eyelids.

Papillae Small, nipple-shaped elevations or projections; raised areas on the tongue in which most of the taste buds are located.

Paralysis Loss or impairment of motor or sensory functions; the inability to move some part of the body voluntarily.

Paralysis agitans A form of Parkinson's disease, of unknown cause.

Parietal bone Cranial bone that forms part of the superior and lateral skull.

Parkinson's disease Progressive deterioration of the basal ganglia in the cerebrum, resulting in diminished production of the neurotransmitter chemical dopamine; causes tremor and slowing of the voluntary skeletal muscle movement and muscle weakness.

Paraplegia Paralysis from the waist down; always involves both legs.

Parasympathetic neurons Part of the autonomic system, originate in ganglia located in the walls of visceral organs; preganglionic fibers come from the brain and the sacral region of the spinal cord.

Patellar reflex Knee-jerk reflex, elicited by striking the knee just below the kneecap (patella).

Peduncles   Stemlike structures that attach the cerebellum to the cerebrum, medulla, and spinal cord.

Perilymph   Fluid that surrounds the sacs in the inner ear.

Peripheral nervous system (PNS)   Portion of the nervous system consisting of nerves and ganglia outside the brain and spinal cord.

Peripheral neuropathy   Damage to the peripheral nerves; can be caused by chronic disorders, by a deficiency of vitamin B_{12}, by taking certain drugs, or from overexposure to toxic substances; symptoms occur gradually. In some cases, its cause is unknown.

Phagocytosis   Process of engulfing and digesting; for example, neuroglia phagocytose bacteria and foreign substances that attack the neurons.

Phantom pain   Sensation of pain seemingly felt in a limb although that limb has been amputated.

Photophobia   Sensitivity to light; abnormal visual intolerance to light, fear of light.

Pia mater   Innermost layer of the meninges, which cover the brain and spinal cord.

Pink eye   See Conjunctivitis.

Pinna   Flap of skin and cartilage that forms the outside portion of the ear.

Plexus   A network of smaller nerves.

Polio   See Poliomyelitis.

Poliomyelitis   A viral infection of the anterior horns of the spinal nerves resulting in destruction of motor neurons that leads to paralysis in the disease's most serious form; also known as polio.

Pons   The middle section of the brain stem; between the medulla oblongata and the midbrain, ventral to the cerebellum.

Posterior median sulcus   See Dorsal median sulcus.

Posterior root   See Dorsal root.

Postganglionic fibers   Nerve fibers that leave the ganglia on either side of the spinal cord.

Postsynaptic neuron   The neuron that is activated by the release of a neurotransmitter substance from another neuron and carries action potentials away from the synapse.

Prefrontal area   Area of the cerebral cortex that controls complex intellectual activities and behavior.

Preganglionic fibers   Nerve fibers that lead to ganglia on either side of the spinal cord.

Premotor area   Area of the cerebral cortex that coordinates large autonomic skeletal muscle activity.

Presbyopia   A hardening and loss of elasticity in the lens of the eye due to advancing age, with resulting inability to focus clearly on near objects.

Presenile dementia   See Alzheimer's disease.

Presynaptic neuron   The neuron that carries an impulse or action potential toward the synapse.

Primary motor area   Area of the cerebral cortex that controls voluntary, fine movements and precise muscle contractions.

Processes   Projections that extend out from the cell body of the neuron.

Proprioreceptors   A receptor located in muscles, tendons and joints that provides information bout body position and movement.

Pupil   Opening in the center of the iris, which contracts and dilates to control the amount of light entering the eye.

Pyramidal pathway   Pathway by which voluntary muscle movements travel from the motor cortex to the spinal cord and then to the effector.

Q

Quadriplegia   Paralysis of all four limbs.

R

REM   See Rapid eye movement sleep.

Rabies   A viral infection of the central nervous system spread by the bite of infected animals.

Radial keratotomy   Series of radiating incisions of the cornea to reduce its curvature.

Radiologic examination   X-rays.

Radiopaque contrast media   Dyes that show up on X-rays.

Rapid eye movement sleep   A state of sleep characterized by symmetrical flutter of the eyes and eyelids, usually associated with dreaming and brain waves similar to those of an awake person (as recorded by an EEG).

Receptor   A specialized cell or nerve cell terminal modified to respond to some specific sense, such as touch, pressure, cold, light, or sound.

Referred pain   Pain that is felt in an area other than the internal organ in which it occurs.

Reflex arc   The most basic conduction pathway through the nervous system, connecting a receptor and an effector.

Refraction   Bending of light as it passes through the structures and fluids of the eye.

Remission   Period without symptoms during the course of a disease.

Resting potential   Balance between positively charged ions on the outside of the nerve cell membrane and negatively charged ions on the inside.

Reticular activating system   System in the brain that controls sleep and wakefulness.

Reticular formation   See Reticular activating system.

Retina   Inner layer of the eyeball, which includes photoreceptors called rods and cones.

Retinal detachment   A complete or partial separation of the retina from the choroid, causing gradual loss of vision.

Retinal vessel occlusion   A disorder in which the artery that supplies blood to the retina or the vein that drains it becomes blocked; causes full or partial blindness if artery is blocked, blurred vision if vein is blocked.

Retinene Vitamin A derivative that is a component of rhodopsin, which is found in the retinal rods.

Reye's syndrome A disease which commonly occurs after an infections illness and causes encephalopathy and cerebral edema.

Rhodopsin Light-sensitive pigment in the retinal rods that stimulates retinal sensory endings; sometimes called visual purple.

Rods Specialized cells in the retina that are sensitive to light.

S

Saccule Smaller of the two sacs in the vestibule.

Sacral nerve Five pairs of spinal nerves that emerge between the sacral vertebrae.

Sacral plexus Network of small nerves that serve the sacral area.

Saltatory conduction Nerve impulse transmission in which the impulse jumps from node to node.

Schwann's cells Tiny, flat cells of the peripheral nervous system that wrap around a nerve fiber jellyroll fashion; they form the neurilemma and the myelin sheath.

Sciatica Pinched or inflamed sciatic nerve, which innervates the legs.

Sclera Tough white exterior coating of the eyeball.

Scleritis Inflammation of the sclera; may occur alone or along with rheumatoid arthritis or digestive tract disorders.

Scotopsin A component of rhodopsin found in the retinal rods.

Seizures Convulsions caused by electrical abnormalities in the brain.

Second lumbar vertebra Bone of the spinal column to which the spinal cord extends.

Semicircular canals Three long canals of the bony inner ear.

Semicircular ducts Tubes within the semicircular canals.

Sensation A state of awareness of external and internal conditions of the body.

Sensorineural hearing loss Hearing loss caused by nerve damage.

Sensory nerve pathways See Afferent nerve pathways.

Sensory nervous system Part of the peripheral nervous system that carries sensations to the spinal cord and brain stem.

Sensory neurons Peripheral neurons that carry impulses from a sense organ to the central nervous system (brain or spinal cord); also called afferent nerve.

Sensory tracts See Ascending tracts.

Serotonin An excitatory neuro-transmitter.

Sharp waves Abnormal EEG wave.

Sheath of Schwann See Neurilemma.

Shingles An acute viral infection of the peripheral nerves; caused by the same virus that causes chickenpox and occurs only in patients who have had chickenpox.

Slow-wave sleep (SWS) See Nonrapid eye movement sleep.

Snellen chart Chart of varying sized letters, used to test vision.

Sodium-potassium pump Mechanism that restores a nerve cell to its resting potential.

Somatic nervous system Part of the peripheral nervous system consisting of the somatic fibers that run between the central nervous system and the skeletal muscles and skin.

Sphenoid nerve Cranial bone at the base of the skull.

Spikes See Sharp waves.

Spinal accessory nerve Cranial nerve (XI) responsible for head and shoulder movement.

Spinal cord A mass of nerve tissue located in the vertebral canal from which 31 pairs of spinal nerves originate.

Spinal puncture See Lumbar puncture.

Spirochete Spiral Shaped bacterium, such as the one that causes Lyme disease.

Spondylosis Abnormal immobility and consolidation of a vertebral joint; also a general term for degenerative changes in the spine.

Stapedectomy Surgical replacement of a rigid stapes with a mobile substitute.

Stapes Tiny stirrup-shaped bone in the middle ear.

Status epilepticus Disorder that causes severe seizures in rapid sequence.

Steroids Medications used to reduce inflammation and swelling.

Stirrup See Stapes.

Strabismus A condition in which the eyes do not focus on an object together; caused by a malalignment of the muscles that control the eyes.

Stroke See Cerebrovascular accident.

Sty An inflammation of one or more of the sebaceous glands of the eyelid.

Subarachnoid space Space between the dura mater and the arachnoid layer and between the arachnoid layer and the pia mater; it is filled with cerebrospinal fluid.

Subdural hematoma Blood clot between the dura mater and the arachnoid layer.

Sulcus Shallow fold in the cerebral cortex.

Superior oblique muscle Muscle that rotates the eyeball downward and outward.

Superior rectus muscle Muscle that moves the eyeball upward and medially.

Sympathetic neurons Part of the autonomic system; they originate in two chains of ganglia on either side of the spinal cord; primarily concerned with processes involving the expenditure of energy.

Sympathetic system   Part of the automatic system that stimulates muscles and glands.

Synapse   A space at the junction between the processes of two neurons; the place where the activity of one neuron affects the activity of another adjacent neuron.

Synaptic cleft   Narrow gap between two neurons.

Syncope   Fainting, brief unconsciousness, caused by an inadequate supply of blood to the brain or cerebral anemia.

T

TIA   See Transient ischemic attack.

Temporal bone   Cranial bone that forms part of the lateral surface and base of the skull.

Terminal ganglia   Ganglia in which parasympathetic neurons originate.

Thalamus   Centers that form most of the tissue of the diencephalon and consist of gray matter.

Theta waves   Abnormal EEG waves.

Thermoreceptor   Receptor stimulated by heat.

Thoracic nerves   Twelve pairs of spinal nerves that emerge between the thoracic vertebrae.

Thoracolumbar system   See Sympathetic system.

Tic douloureux   Painful nervous system disorder that affects the seventh cranial nerve.

Tonometer   Instrument that measures pressure within the eye.

Trabeculae   Tiny extensions that hold the arachnoid membrane above the pia mater.

Transient ischemic attack   A sudden, temporary blockage of a cerebral blood vessel that causes temporary, minor symptoms similar to a stroke; can be a warning sign of an impending stroke.

Tremors   Involuntary movements characteristic of Parkinson's disease.

Trigeminal nerve   Cranial nerve (V) responsible for sensation in the head and face and for chewing.

Trochlear nerve   Cranial nerve (IV) responsible for eyeball movement.

Tympanic membrane   Thin membrane of skin and mucous membrane that separates the middle ear from the outer ear.

U

Unipolar neuron   Having a single pole or process; neuron in which the axon and the dendrite fuse at the cell body and for a short distance beyond; begins as a bipolar neuron, but after the embryonic stage of fetal development it changes.

Utricle   Larger of the two sacs in the vestibule.

V

Vagus nerve   Cranial nerve (X) responsible for sensation and movement in the larynx, trachea, heart, stomach, and other organs.

Vasoconstrictors   Medications that constrict or widen the blood vessels.

Vasodilators   Medications that dilate or widen the blood vessels.

Ventral median fissure   Deep groove on the anterior side of the spinal cord that divides it in half lengthwise.

Ventral ramus (pl. rami)   Branch of the spinal nerve.

Ventral root   Anterior root that attaches each spinal nerve to the spinal cord.

Ventricles   Cavities in the brain.

Vertebrae (pl. vertebra)   A bony separate segment of the spinal column.

Vertebral arteriogram   Angiogram that outlines the vertebral arteries in the neck and the posterior cerebral arteries of the brain.

Vesicle   A tiny sac or bladder containing liquid.

Vestibule   Small chamber that is separated from the middle ear by an oval-shaped "window" of membrane.

Vestibulocochlear nerve   Cranial nerve (VIIII) responsible for hearing and balance.

Viscera   Internal organs.

Vesicle   A tiny sac or bladder containing liquid.

Vitreous body   Transparent gel that fills the space behind the lens of the eye, maintains eyeball shape, and supports the retina.

Vitreous humor   Watery substance in the vitreous body.

Visceral effector   Effector neurons of the autonomic system that control the cardiac muscle, smooth muscle, and glandular tissues.

Visceral system   See Autonomic neurons system.

Visceroreceptor or visceroceptor   Provides information about the body's internal environment.

W

White matter   Bundles of myelinated nerve fibers, which appear white because of the presence of myelin.